Contemporary Nutrition for Latinos

Contemporary Nutrition for Latinos

A Latino Lifestyle Guide to Nutrition and Health

Dr. Judith C. Rodriguez, R.D., F.A.D.A.

iUniverse Star
New York Lincoln Shanghai

Contemporary Nutrition for Latinos
A Latino Lifestyle Guide to Nutrition and Health

iUniverse Star
an iUniverse, Inc. imprint

For information address:
iUniverse, Inc.
2021 Pine Lake Road, Suite 100
Lincoln, NE 68512
www.iuniverse.com

ISBN: 0-595-29730-7

Printed in the United States of America

Many thanks to my husband George, and my family and friends for their encouragement and support. A thank you also goes to Toni Martin, R.D., Maribel Rosario, R.D., Dr. Otilia Salmon, Mr. Francisco Estevez, Blanca Lopez, R.D., Amita Dave, R.D., and others who helped with this manuscript.

Contents

Consult your physician and a Registered/Licensed Dietitian before starting a weight management or special diet program.

Chapter 1
Healthy Eating

Introduction

Yes, most of us love to eat our traditional Latino/Hispanic foods. We delight in sharing our rice and beans, tortillas, *tamales, pasteles, congri, gallo pinto,* and many other favorite dishes with family and friends. But we are just as likely to have non-traditional foods for lunch, such as hamburgers and french fries. On a busy day, we may buy french fries at our favorite local eatery, bring them home, and serve them with a home prepared meal. Even when we eat our traditional foods, we may not prepare them using traditional methods. How many of us make our own seasoning or flavoring bases such as *sofrito,* or prepare our own *adobo?* We often purchase a jar of *recaito, adobo,* and even Mexican *salsa!*

Personally, I prefer to eat in my favorite Latino/Hispanic restaurant when eating out, but my sister-in-law would never do that. She prefers to prepare her own traditional foods. "Why pay for something you can make at home that tastes better?" she asks as if I were crazy. But, she will be dressed in two minutes flat if offered a chance to go to her favorite seafood restaurant. Frequently we enjoy eating foods in our own unique way, by combining home and commercially prepared foods.

How can we combine traditional and new foods, and at the same time ensure that the eating habits that evolve in our families are beneficial? Good health and positive habits are two of the best gifts that we can give our families and other loved ones, our community, and ourselves. With some basic knowledge about nutrition, selection, and preparation of foods, we can meet the challenges for good health that will face us this millennium!

A Guide to the Book's Format

To facilitate reading and utilizing the information in this book, each chapter contains introductory and general information. There are also four sections in almost all the chapters titled Consumer Tips, Issues, Contemporary Latino/Hispanic Life, and Food and Nutrition in This Millennium. The second section, **Consumer Tips,** provides information that will help us select, purchase, and prepare foods. The third section, **Issues,** addresses current, controversial, or contradictory information and concerns. The next section, **Contemporary Latino/Hispanic Life,** provides ideas that may be useful to our daily life, or ideas for combining traditional and new behaviors. The last section, **Food and Nutrition in This Millennium,** discusses trends, changes, and ways we can keep abreast and be prepared for new and changing information.

The chapters in this book cover topics that are of interest and are useful to consumers. The book begins with information on the use and application of food guides (chapter 2); carbohydrates, proteins, and fats (chapter 3); vitamins and minerals (chapter 4); phytochemicals [health promoting chemicals] and herbs (chapter 5); dietary supplements (chapter 6); and suggestions for combining traditional and modern foods (chapter 7).

Did you know that every year over 2000 new food products are introduced? As the modern market provides these new products, it becomes even more important to know what food to buy, and how to buy it. We also need to know about food safety and how to prepare foods in ways that are convenient and maximize nutrients. Chapter 8 discusses shopping and labeling, and provides tips for selecting, preparing, and storing foods.

Obesity is a major health problem for Latinos and/or Hispanics, as well as the general United States population. A large contributor to childhood and adult obesity are eating high calorie meals and snacks, and eating out (especially during holiday seasons). Therefore, chapter 9 covers key health concerns, nutrient needs throughout the life cycle, and tips for choosing healthy foods for different age groups. Chapter 10 provides basic weight management information and provides tips for selecting a sound weight management plan.

Many Latinos and/or Hispanics suffer from diabetes, hypertension (high blood pressure), heart disease, and the other illnesses common in contemporary societies. Of the top ten diseases in the United States, at least six can be avoided or controlled through diet. How we manage our health (or disease condition) will have a strong impact on our quality of life. Chapter 11 covers major diet-related diseases and gives tips for their dietary management. Chapter 12 provides tips for selecting nutritious snacks, and eating healthy both during the holidays and when eating out. The last chapter (chapter 13) provides some sample menus for different situations.

Beginning a new century fills us with a sense of renewal, opportunity, hope, and enthusiasm. What better way to live it than in good health?

CONSUMER TIPS

The Influence of Advertising

Do you know a particular person that believes he or she "must have" a particular brand of cheese, sneakers, or other product because of its perceived status? Advertising is a common part of our modern, everyday life. Written, radio, and television ads provide us with information concerning available products. Advertising encourages us to use a particular product from the wide variety available. Ads can also create a false sense of need or self worth from the acquisition of unnecessary products. We may buy particular foods because they represent an aspired status, or we identify them with a particular lifestyle. When selecting an item, ask yourself:

1. Why do I want this product?
2. Is my need for this product physiological, social, or emotional?
3. Is there a lower priced equivalent? If so, why am I rejecting it?
4. Can I do without this product?
5. Can I, and am I willing to, make this product instead of buying it?
6. Is the information that I am receiving about this product influencing me to purchasing it, or am I using the information to make a wise choice?

Product manufacturers have "discovered" the Latino/Hispanic consumer market. Latinos/Hispanics have a purchasing power of over 350 billion dollars a year. Companies want our dollars and our loyalty to their products. Brand loyalty means that we use a product unquestioningly or without comparison shopping. But is it more important for us to choose and eat foods that both taste good and are healthy.

What We Eat Is a Choice, Not a Chance

Change from fatalistic thinking to empowered behavior! Empowered behavior means that we find out about, make decisions, and take actions to care for our health.

Identify opportunities to make choices. Many persons tell me that they do not eat well because their lifestyle does not give them that chance. But an important part of success with our goals is to plan for the chaos, so that what we eat becomes a choice, not a chance. Planning for chaos also helps to minimize the chances for a relapse. This is key in making a successful change.

What are your most "chaotic" times during the day? How does this influence what you eat? For example, midday is a chaotic time for many of us, especially if we are working outside the home. As a result, we may skip meals or eat poorly. How should we manage this chaos? First, remember that it is easier to plan what to eat during chaotic times than to try to change the chaos.

Knowing that we have planned something to eat helps to reduce the stress. Why not plan on things that are important to your health, such as exercising, preparing a healthy snack, or relaxing?

This will give you the satisfaction of using your time wisely and effectively. We deserve *to give ourselves the best care and health* possible.

The Gift of Good Health

Have you heard the saying, "It's not the size of the gift that counts?" Good health is a gift that cannot be seen and is not obvious for many years. It is one of the best gifts that you can give your family. In many cases, your family will not even be aware of this "secret gift." Not only will you improve your overall health, you will also influence your children's health through positive behavior. They will have the advantage of having learned and adopted positive habits early in life instead of later having to change the negative behaviors to positive behaviors. Your children will also learn that great gifts of love are not money or material things, but the positive things that you have taught them. What a wonderful gift!

ISSUES

Health of Latinos/Hispanics

Our traditional toast says *"salud, dinero, y amor"* (health, money, and love). Have you noticed that (good) health is the first wish of good fortune? Latinos/Hispanics know that with good health we can seek out other fortunes. Money and love will be harder to achieve in the absence of good health. But, in trying to keep up with our busy modern lives, we often forget about, or neglect, our health.

The common illnesses among people living in contemporary societies are heart disease, diabetes, cancer, dental disease, adult bone loss, and obesity. Latinos/Hispanics have a high incidence of type 2 diabetes, obesity, dental disease, and hypertension. The prevalence of hypertension is higher in men than in women. A large number of Latinos/Hispanics have a higher than desirable blood cholesterol level. Alcohol plays a part in three other health concerns: accidents, suicides, and chronic liver disease (cirrhosis).

Although Latinos/Hispanics are at a lower risk for the more common types of cancers affecting the overall US population, cancer is still the second leading cause of death in US Latinos/Hispanics after heart disease. About 60% of cancer deaths are related to environmental factors and lifestyle, which includes diet. But, we can reduce our cancer risk by adding more fresh fruits and vegetables to our diets. For example, we can substitute the colas with juice, and eat meats that are low in fat and calories.

In addition to diet, lifestyle factors that impact health are:

• Sleep
• Stress
• Environmental quality
• Smoking and the use of other tobacco products
• Alcohol consumption or other substance abuse
• Lack of sufficient exercise or physical activity

Are any of these lifestyle factors affecting your health or putting you at risk for illness or disease? It is difficult to imagine that anyone living in today's contemporary society is not faced with at least two or three of these risk factors. It is hard to find someone that is getting enough sleep or does not feel stressed!

Nutrition and Health

Nutrition refers to the taking in of food to support growth, renewal, maintenance, and repair of the body. **Overnutrition** refers to eating too much of all or some foods and may include little or no exercise. Being overweight and obese are imbalances between the calories you eat and the calories you use. Slow metabolism (thyroid imbalance) may be responsible for only a small percentage of obesity.

Undernutrition refers to a lack of enough food or nutrients and its physical, mental, and social consequences. This undernutrition can be externally imposed, such as in the lack of available food. It can be internally imposed, such as in the person that has been following an extremely low calorie diet for the purposes of weight loss or because of an illness. It is very difficult to get the needed nutrients when eating a low calorie diet.

Young girls who want a "model's" figure may diet to dangerous levels. Throughout the United States and Latin America, young girls are dieting at earlier and earlier ages. Although these behaviors are more common in females, they also occur in males. Some athletes also attempt extreme dieting regimens.

This exaggerated concern with weight can develop into eating disorders such as anorexia or bulimia. A person with *anorexia* may refuse to eat, exercise compulsively, have other harmful behaviors, and experience extreme weight loss. A person with *bulimia* secretly eats enormous amounts of food and abuses laxatives or induces vomiting in attempts to maintain a desired weight or figure. These behaviors require intervention and help. Do not wait to intervene. Get your loved one to seek professional help immediately!

Imbalances of nutrient intakes can also cause malnutrition. For example, diet related iron-deficiency anemia may occur when a person does not eat enough foods containing iron. Sometimes a person may take excessive amounts of a mineral or vitamin pills. The easy availability and consumption of concentrated levels of nutrients or other substances in pill form promotes excessive intake and can cause a nutritional imbalance. As a result, the person becomes malnourished or ill from excessive intake of the nutrient. It is wise to remember that neither too little nor too much is "healthy."

CONTEMPORARY LATINO/HISPANIC LIFE

Preparing for Change

Do you live to eat or eat to live? Let's face it—our modern life is surrounded by food. We live with the contradiction of controlling what we eat in the midst of food abundance. Can you eat less without feeling deprived?

We can minimize the impact of some risk factors by not partaking in activities such as smoking, excessive alcohol consumption, or substance abuse. But we must change and learn to manage activities, such as stress, insufficient exercise, or lack of sleep. You will not make any changes in your food habits unless you believe that you *need* to change, and that if you do, the change will be a *benefit*, not a *deprivation*.

Ask yourself the following:

- Do my appearance and my health matter to me?
- For what conditions am I most at risk? Being overweight? Heart disease? High blood pressure? Diabetes?
- What lifestyle and genetic factors make me susceptible?
- What can I do?
- What and how do I stand to benefit from these positive changes?
- Am I willing to make these changes?
- Do I have the knowledge and skills needed to make these changes?
- What must I do to get the needed knowledge and skills?

Remember that although making the changes cannot guarantee freedom from illness, the changes can reduce your risk. Should you become ill, a good health status and positive health habits will help you manage an illness, which affects your quality of life.

Defining and Refining "Eating Habits"

It will be up to each of us to develop an identity that combines the traditional with the modern. Some of us will want to emphasize traditional values or combine them with our modern lifestyle. In either case, a big part of how *your* goal is achieved is through the eating habits that you develop.

Determine your values and goals. Identify the foods and behaviors that move you toward your values and goals. Don't be afraid to use *traditional and modern foods.* After all, it is very difficult and unlikely that we can be pure traditionalists or modernists.

Ask yourself some of the following questions:

- Do I want to emphasize the **traditional food habits** that are unique to my country of ancestry?

- Do I want to emphasize a cuisine that reflects a **combination** of United States and ancestral roots (for example, a combination of common U.S. and Colombian foods)?

- Do I want to move toward a "**fusion**" (Nuevo Latino) cuisine that reflects the various Latin American influences in the U.S. (for example, a combination of Mexican, Cuban, and Puerto Rican cuisine)?

- Do I want to move toward an **international cuisine** (for example Latin American, Asian, Middle Eastern, and European cuisine)?

After you have determined your own "**culture of eating,**" begin to identify healthy foods that reflect that culture. Determine how much you want to emphasize and combine eating traditional and/or modern foods. For example, if you want to eat an international cuisine, identify how to get some of your nutrients and phytochemicals from a combination of traditional Latino and Chinese vegetables, such as a *sancocho* or other thick stews that also includes Chinese cabbage.

Readiness and Willingness to Change

Another point to consider is your readiness or willingness to change. We are all at different stages of change for each of our health goals. If you can identify your stage of change, it is easier to work on your goals. Identify a nutrition-related issue. Use the chart below to determine your "stage of change" by finding one example that best fits your readiness level. I have given you an example in the middle column.

Readiness Level	Example/Issue: Fats	Your Issue:
You haven't really thought about it	You haven't really thought about eating less fat	
You are starting to think about it	You are thinking that maybe you should eat less fat	
You have started or are making some changes	You have started eating less fat by putting less butter on your bread	
You have made changes but occasionally go back to the "old" habit	You now try to avoid fried foods and use low fat milk but still eat more fried foods than you want to	
You have managed to make changes and stick to them	You try to limit fried foods to no more than once every two weeks	

Once you know "where you are at," think of ways that you can strengthen that level. Next, ask yourself how you can move on to the next level until you have reached your goal. Plan your steps one by one. Give yourself time. If you "fall back," start again!

Making changes in the way you eat will take a long time. You have probably had these habits for many years, so it will take time to learn new ones. The key is **practice, practice, practice!**

Make Healthy Eating Your Habit of Choice

Remember, to make a change permanent, it must become a habit. Make the new change an automatic behavior and a part of your life. Practice the behavior every chance you get, until you find yourself doing it without having to "think about it." When you suddenly find yourself asking for water or juice with your meal instead of soda, you will realize that your positive behavior is now a habit!

Food and Nutrition in This Millennium

In this millennium, the only constant will be change. We will not survive life's challenges and grow without strong cultural roots, and a healthy body and mind. Knowledge and understanding about our health and cultural strengths, the positive values and behaviors, will give us strong roots. The ability to obtain new information, face challenges, and make healthy food choices will help us grow strong and face the inevitability of change in good health, wisdom, and dignity.

Chapter 2

Food Guides

Understanding and Using Food Guides

What is a Food Plan?

A food plan is a guide for healthy eating. A guide is divided into groups of foods. A guide provides information about **each food group,** the foods that "fit" into that group, the **recommended serving sizes,** and the **recommended number of servings.** Many food guides include a picture or model (such as a pyramid) that makes it easier for a person to learn and remember the guidelines.

The most common food plan or guide used in the United States is the **Food Guide Pyramid,** developed by the United States Department of Agriculture. This plan provides general guidelines for the *healthy* population with no special dietary needs. Other commonly used guides are the **Mediterranean Diet Pyramid** and the **Latin American Diet Pyramid,** available at www.oldwayspt.org. Infants, persons on special diets, and physically active people need special plans.

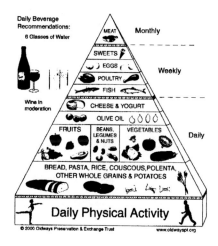

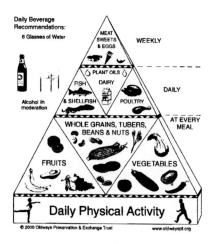

Food Guide Pyramid
A Guide to Daily Food Choices

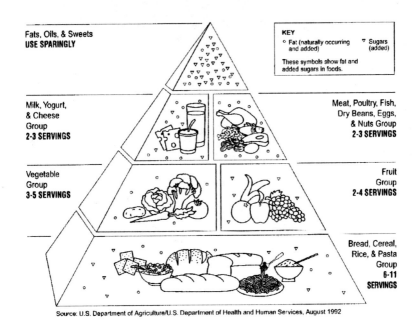

Fats, Oils, & Sweets
USE SPARINGLY

KEY
○ Fat (naturally occurring and added)   ▽ Sugars (added)
These symbols show fat and added sugars in foods.

Milk, Yogurt, & Cheese Group
2-3 SERVINGS

Meat, Poultry, Fish, Dry Beans, Eggs, & Nuts Group
2-3 SERVINGS

Vegetable Group
3-5 SERVINGS

Fruit Group
2-4 SERVINGS

Bread, Cereal, Rice, & Pasta Group
6-11 SERVINGS

Source: U.S. Department of Agriculture/U.S. Department of Health and Human Services, August 1992

Breads, cereals, rice, pasta, and other grains

Notice that in the United States' Food Guide Pyramid, breads, cereals, rice, pasta, and other grains are recommended as the **basic or core foods** that provide calories (energy) in our diet. It is recommended that we eat 6-11 servings a day. We generally consume enough of these foods throughout the day, and do not even realize it. For example, we may have bread with our coffee, or cereal in the morning, and bread (as part of a sandwich) for lunch, crackers for a snack, and a large serving of rice or a few tortillas (which may count as two or more servings) at dinnertime.

Fruits and vegetables

The next important groups of foods are fruits and vegetables. These foods provide many different vitamins, minerals, fiber and phytochemicals, which seem to have disease protection qualities. So it is recommended that we eat five *or more* servings a day. Many of our traditional diets include a lot of fruits or juices as snacks, and vegetables in our mixed dishes and stews. Since we are eating more non-traditional foods, many of us may now be eating fewer fruits and vegetables. We need to make a greater effort to eat more of these foods.

Milk and milk products

We need to drink skim or low fat milk and eat milk products such as cheese and yogurt, because they provide important nutrients such as calcium and protein. About two to four servings are recommended per day. Nowadays many children are drinking soda or other sugared beverages with meals or snacks instead of milk. As a result, they may not be getting enough calcium.

Many adults do not drink enough milk because "it bothers them" or they believe that they do not need it. If milk "bothers" you, that is, causes gas, pain, or diarrhea, drink **lactose** free or "**low in lactose**." milk. Cheeses and yogurt are good alternatives. You need the calcium and other nutrients that are in these dairy products, so try to eat enough of them throughout the day.

Meats and meat substitutes

The meat and meat substitutes group includes meat, fish, poultry, beans, eggs, and nuts. It is recommended that we have about 2-3 servings a day. Sometimes we eat meat and beans at the same meal. This equals two portions, so it can be easy to eat too much of this group.

Other foods: fats, oils, and sweets

The fats, oils, and sweets are placed at the small peak on top of the Food Guide Pyramid to remind us that these foods are not basic, and should be eaten sparingly. These foods are used as accents and/or flavors. However, many of us are eating too many foods from this group. These foods can add many extra calories to our diet without giving us many nutrients. For example, the sugar we add to our coffee, the sugar in presweetened cereals and the butter or margarine on our bread can add hundreds of calories to our diet.

If we drink a soda and eat a candy bar, more sugar and fat will have been added to the day's diet. Later, we may eat French Fries, a piece of fried chicken, dressing in the salad, or butter on the bread. Just imagine—we will have had more than nine servings of fats, oils, and sweets in one day! That is probably **more** servings from this group than any other food group in the Food Guide Pyramid.

Other Food Plans

Many places or countries, for example, Guatemala or Mexico, use plans designed for their populations. These food plans may or may not be in the shape of a Food Guide Pyramid, but their purpose is the same: to provide the population with easy to remember guidelines for healthy eating.

For example, in the United States, the Food Guide Pyramid includes starchy vegetables in the "vegetables" group. But the *Pirámide de Alimentos de Puerto Rico* includes starchy vegetables, or the *viandas,* with the "bread, cereals, and other grains" group. Neither of these guides are wrong, they are just based on the common use of the foods in their area or a population.

Some groups or persons may modify a food plan for specific purposes. For example, vegetarians may develop a food guide pyramid with a "meat substitutes" group. Or, a food company that produces canned foods may develop a pyramid with pictures of its products.

There are also food guides for special populations. Persons with diabetes commonly use a guide called the "diabetic exchange lists." Other food guides are designed for persons on weight control diets, or individuals with heart or kidney disease.

Understanding and Using Food Guides

So, why spend so much time explaining different food guides? It is because throughout the years, I have found that this is a common area of confusion among many persons.

Do not be confused if the following happens: you attend a lecture on healthy eating and are advised to plan your meals using the Food Guide Pyramid. You are told that potatoes and corn are in the "vegetables" group, and breads are in the "grains" group. Then, you attend another lecture with your spouse, who has type 2 diabetes, on planning meals, and are told that potatoes and corn are in the "starches" group, which also includes breads.

Don't worry. It means that the advice given to you was based on food guides with specific objectives. For example, remember that the Food Guide Pyramid is for healthy persons. For persons with diabetes, the goal of the food plan is to regulate carbohydrate intake, so foods are grouped according to how much carbohydrates they contain.

There are many types of plans available, and different ones are used depending on the individual's need. It is important that you know your needs so that you use the appropriate food guide.

CONSUMER TIPS

You can easily and quickly evaluate what you eat with a food record. Write down the foods you ate in one day and see if you ate the amounts recommended in each food group. Here is an example:

Sample of an Analysis of a Food Record for One Meal						
Foods You Ate	Grains & Substitutes (6-11)	Fruits (2-3)	Vegetables (2-3)	Milk & Substitutes (2-4)	Meats & Substitutes (2)	Other (Sparingly)
Congri or *Gallo Pinto* (1 ½ cups, total)	2 (about 1 cup of rice)				½ serving (about ½ cup of black beans)	
Fried Eggs (2)					1 serving (2 eggs are one serving)	1 (oil for frying the eggs)
Fruit Shake: (1/2 cup *mamey* puree, 1/2 cup milk, sugar)		1 (1/2 cup *mamey* puree)		½ (1/2 cup milk)		1 (sugar)
Totals	2 of 6-11	1 of 2-3	0 of 2-3	½ of 2-4	1 ½ of 2	2

Notice: This meal included fat (oil) and sugar but no vegetables. In this example, a person can "balance" the next meal by including **vegetables,** some more **grains, fruit,** and **dairy.** Only a little bit more meat or meat substitutes is needed. It would be better to avoid fats and sugar the next meal.

Suggestions for the next meal

- **At home**—a thick soup or stew (*sancocho* or *asopado),* with lots of vegetables, and a small amount of meat about the size of your thumb. Have it with bread, a small piece of cheese, and a glass of orange juice.

• **Eating** out—spaghetti with marinara sauce and grated cheese, a side salad, and orange juice or a fruit salad as the dessert.

Evaluate Your Intake						
Foods You Ate	Grains & Substitutes (6 - 11)	Fruits (2-3)	Vegetables (2-3)	Dairy Products (2-4)	Meat & Substitutes (2)	Other (In Moderation)
Total						

After you have kept a record of all the foods you ate in one day (24 hours), total the number of servings from each group. It is best if you do this for several (four to seven) days and get an average. The data will provide an overall estimate of how you ate during the week.

Check for the following:

1. Were you low (below the recommended amounts) for any food groups? Which one(s)?

2. Were you over the recommended amounts for any food groups? Which one(s)?

3. How could you have easily changed your choices to be closer to the recommended amounts?

Find **easy** ways to improve your eating habits. For example, if you are low in fruits or dairy, perhaps you can replace the soda with juice, milk, or have a shake made with banana and milk.

Estimating Food Group Servings in Mixed Dishes

Some common Latino/Hispanic dishes include many food groups, depending on how we prepare them. We can estimate how much of a serving of a food group is in a mixed dish.

For example, remember, 1 egg is 1/2 of a recommended meat serving. If you make a *Flan* with eight eggs for eight servings, each serving will contain one half serving from the meat group. You may also "count" about one serving from the dairy group, if you prepare the *Flan* with undiluted evaporated milk. *Note:* If you prepare the *Flan* with condensed milk, we cannot count this as a milk serving because it does not contain enough milk to be considered a milk serving.

Substitutions to Improve Food Intakes and Make Dishes More Nutritious

You can also make small recipe changes in dishes to make them more nutritious. For example, here are some simple substitutions that you can make in a *Flan*:

- Many *Flan* recipes use 4 cans of **condensed** milk. Use 4 cans of **undiluted evaporated milk** instead. Add sugar to taste, about 1 1/2 cups. This will give you much more calcium!

- If you are on a diet, have a smaller serving of *Flan*, or use **undiluted evaporated skim milk** in the recipe.

- Replace some of the whole egg with egg whites. Use 2 egg whites in place of 1 egg. You can also use low cholesterol egg substitutes.

Ingredient Substitutions in *Flan*

Usual ingredient	Substitution	
	Low Fat	High Calcium
Eggs	Use egg whites or egg substitutes	
Condensed milk		Use undiluted evaporated skim milk

ISSUES

Yes, Our Foods Fit into All Food Plans!

When I worked in a clinic that served many Latinos, a frequent comment from my clients was that it was difficult to eat well because our food did not fit into the Food Guides. But our foods do fit into food plans, including the Food Guide Pyramid!

When traditional and new foods are properly combined, the Latino diet can be very health promoting. The key is to know which foods are the better choices, the amounts, and where the foods fit!

Some examples of common foods and their corresponding food group in the Food Guide Pyramid are:

- Grains—tortillas (flour or corn), rice, *masa harina,* cornstarch, oatmeal
- Fruits—mango, pineapple, banana, oranges
- Vegetables—potatoes, salsa or tomato sauce, yams, lettuce, sweet potato, corn
- Milk and milk substitutes—low fat milk, skim milk, cheese
- Meat—fish, chicken, beans, eggs, tofu, or soybeans

- Other (fats and sugars)—olives, olive oil, corn oil, cream cheese, sour cream, coconut, bacon, lard, sugar. Remember to eat these infrequently and always in small amounts.

Many Latino dishes are combination dishes. That means that we are eating different groups of foods from the Food Guide Pyramid in one dish.

For example, a taco may contain:

- One serving from the grain group (corn tortilla)
- One serving from the meat and meat substitutes group (beans or meat)
- One serving from the vegetable group (lettuce, chopped tomatoes, onions, and salsa)
- About one-third serving from the milk and milk substitutes group (shredded cheese)
- About one serving of "other." Remember, hard tortillas are usually fried, giving us extra fat and calories.

A taco is generally a good combination dish if we make it with lean meat or beans, a small amount of cheese, and lots of lettuce, onion, tomatoes, and salsa. Drink it with a **glass of skim milk**, which increases the dairy group serving, or a **glass of orange juice**, to include a fruit serving.

CONTEMPORARY LATINO/HISPANIC LIFE

Water is the Most Important Nutrient in Our Diet

Are you too busy to drink water? Do you think about water when you think about nutrition? Although water provides no calories, it is the most important nutrient! We can go without some nutrients for weeks or months before we develop a deficiency, but we cannot live without water for more than just a few days! One of my favorite food guides is the Puerto Rican Food Guide Pyramid, because it is one of the few food guides that includes water.

Human beings are about 60% water. So, if you weigh 140 lbs. (64 kg) about 84 lbs. (38 kg.) of you is water. Water protects body organs. It dissolves and moves some substances throughout the body. Water makes many important reactions possible. Water has many other important functions, among them the regulation of body temperature.

We should drink about *8 glasses of fluids* throughout the day, and *most* of it should be water. For example, we can have a cup of coffee at breakfast time; a glass of water midmorning; a glass of orange juice and a glass of water with lunch, a glass of milk and a glass of water in the afternoon; a glass of apple juice at dinnertime, and a glass of water in the evening. This will give us our eight (8) glasses a day.

Drink water regularly throughout the day. It does not have to be fancy, expensive, bottled water. Tap water that is safe to drink is fine. If you are not sure it is safe, boil it and put it in your refrigerator. Water is healthy, has no calories, helps clean our mouth, and washes away cavity-forming bacteria. Clean, safe, tap water is cheaper than soda!

If you wait until you are thirsty to drink water, you have waited too long. Thirst is not triggered until our body has lost about 1-2% of its total body water. It is *very* important for infants, the elderly, and persons that live in hot and/or humid areas to drink plenty of water.

Suggestions for Water Replacement

- Be careful to drink enough water on hot and humid days and before and after physical activity.

- Weigh yourself before and after exercise or other physical activity. Drink 2 glasses of water for every pound lost during exercise.

- Drink water, not alcoholic beverages or beverages that contain caffeine as these stimulate urination (water loss).

- If you drink juice after exercise, dilute it with water. Otherwise you may drink more calories than you used up!

- You don't need special sports drinks. If you want them, drink them only if you are doing vigorous exercise for two or more hours. The drink should have about 5-10% carbohydrates, and have about equal amounts of sodium and potassium. (Juices have about 10-15% carbohydrates and sports drinks have about 5-8 % carbohydrates. You can dilute your juice by adding an equal amount of water).

- Eat fruit only after you have had water. Fruit alone may satisfy your taste buds but not provide enough replacement fluids.

Alcoholic Beverages—Do They Fit In Your Diet?

The keys to alcohol consumption are *social context* (as when having a meal with friends) and *moderation*. Wine, beer, and other alcoholic beverages provide calories, but little or no nutritional value. In excess, alcohol can be harmful because it becomes toxic to your organs and replaces nutritious foods.

But many of us like to drink a glass of wine with, or after, a meal. If you drink, the general recommendation is a maximum of one drink per day for women, and two for men. About 12 ounces of beer, 1 1/2 ounces of 80 proof alcohol, or 5 ounces of wine have the same amount of alcohol. Drinking coffee does not make the intoxication go away.

Some suggestions are:

- If you don't drink, don't start.

- Only drink alcohol accompanied by foods or after you have eaten.

- Once you have had one or two drinks, switch to water or calorie-free beverages.

Common Errors Concerning Fats

Probably the most common error people make related to using the Food Guide Pyramid has to do with fats. Butter, margarine, oil, cream cheese, olives, avocado, coconut, bacon, pork rinds, chicken skins, fried chicken skins, and dressings are high in fat and belong in the "Other" group of the Food Guide Pyramid.

Making a Food Plan Fit Your Cultural Heritage and Lifestyle

A food guide helps us identify categories of foods that need emphasis and groups that may need to be consumed less. For Latinos/Hispanics, I have found that the meat and meat substitutes and the "Other" groups are the groups from which many of us eat the most. For example, coffee with sugar, sodas, and fried foods. We may not vary our diet enough or eat enough from the milk, fruit, and vegetable groups. If that sounds like you, try some of the following:

• Skip meat when you serve beans.

• Sprinkle some parmesan or grated cheese over the salad or the beans.

• Add chopped carrots or chopped pumpkin to the beans.

• Cook or prepare your favorite rice dishes with small amounts of mixed vegetables.

• Include a small salad with meals.

• Drink low fat or skim milk or juice instead of soda.

• Mix equal parts juice and water with artificial sweetener to make a juice drink.

If you are trying to save time, combine convenience (pre-prepared foods) with home prepared foods. For example, some families purchase prepared roasted chicken and make the rice and salad once they get home. As you can see, with good planning, both traditional and non-traditional foods can easily fit into your lifestyle and food and nutrition related goals.

Food and Nutrition in This Millennium

It is likely that the Food Guide Pyramid and other models will continue to change to include new foods or information. Some possible changes include:

- emphasis on eating more fruits, vegetables, and different grains;
- emphasis on the calcium-enriched and low fat dairy products;
- emphasis on eating more meat substitutes, such as beans and tofu (soybeans);
- increased popularity or use of the Latin American Food Guide or the Mediterranean Food Guide Pyramid, or other pyramids and styles of eating that include eating many more fruits, vegetables, grains, legumes, and fish, the use of olive oil, an occasional serving of wine, and fewer or lean cuts meats;
- eating more convenient, nutritionally enhanced (functional) foods;
- eating more sugar substitutes or fat substitutes and food supplements, and
- increased physical activity along with healthy food choices.

Chapter 3
Carbohydrates, Proteins, and Fats

Food, Calories and You

Calories are a measure of the amount of energy in a food. A high calorie food provides us with a lot of energy. Because we need energy every day, it is important to eat. Some energy containing nutrients form what is known as blood sugar (blood glucose). This blood glucose gives our body the energy it needs to function, breathe, and perform all other activities, just like gasoline is needed for a car.

The calories in our foods are a "problem" only if we are eating more food than we need. If we take in more calories than we are using up, the body stores these extra calories as glycogen (body starch) or fat. This causes us to become overweight.

What Provides Calories?

We get our calories (also called energy) from carbohydrates, proteins, and fats. We also get calories from alcohol. Energy in the form of alcohol is not utilized well, and too much can be harmful to the body. That is why we do not consider alcohol a nutrient.

How Many Calories?		
Calorie Source	Calories Per Gram	Calories Per Level Teaspoon (4 Grams)
Carbohydrate	4	16
Protein	4	16
Alcohol	7	28
Fat	9	36

Per gram, carbohydrates and proteins provide four calories, and alcohol provides seven calories. Fats provide nine calories. This is *more than twice* the calories of carbohydrates and proteins!

Carbohydrates

Carbohydrates are one of the most important nutrients in our daily diet. Yet, many people mistakenly believe that carbohydrates are "bad" foods. What are some myths and truths about carbohydrates?

Myth	Truth
Carbohydrates are fattening.	• Carbohydrates have fewer calories than fats. • Too many calories (no matter the source) will make us gain weight.
Sugars cause diabetes.	• Sugar does not cause diabetes. • There are three types of diabetes, and the cause is insufficient or no production of a hormone called insulin. • Insulin helps the body use blood glucose. • Regulating carbohydrate intake, especially the sugars, helps to manage diabetes.
Carbohydrates should not be eaten when dieting.	• Carbohydrates give us energy, so we need them for our daily activities. • If we do not eat enough carbohydrates, we break down our muscle protein and use it for energy. • Eating enough carbohydrates prevents the breaking down of muscle protein, so we need carbohydrates even when we are trying to lose weight. • The key is to avoid eating too many carbohydrates or total calories.

Carbohydrates should be our primary choice of energy. They are the energy used by our body, including the brain. Fat is not the source of energy normally used by the brain because it has other important functions. Protein is most important for making and repairing tissues, not providing energy.

Types of carbohydrates

There are two main types of carbohydrates, the *simple* carbohydrates and the *complex* carbohydrates. Simple carbohydrate is the term used to describe different types of sugars. Complex carbohydrates is the term used to describe different types of starches and dietary fibers.

Simple Carbohydrates		
Name	**What It Is**	**Sources**
Glucose	This is the sugar used for energy by the body. It is also known as blood glucose or dextrose.	It is found in animals (including humans) and plants. All the sugars and starches that we eat become blood glucose and are used by the body. If we do not use glucose, it is changed to fat and stored.
Fructose	This is the sugar that is found naturally in fruits and vegetables (as in sweet corn).	May be purchased as a sweetener. Commercial fructose is usually made from cornstarch, not extracted from fruits.
Sucrose	Common table sugar, made from sugar cane or beet sugar.	Available in many forms: sugar, brown sugar, powdered sugar, sugar cubes, turbinado sugar, raw sugar.
Lactose	The sugar in milk.	Not generally available commercially.
Honey	Sugar formed from the nectar gathered by bees. It is made up of water, sucrose, fructose, and glucose.	The source of the honey determines its name. **Do not** give honey to infants because germs in it may cause illness and even death.
Complex Carbohydrates (Starches)		
Name	**What It Is**	**Sources**
Starches	Long chains of sugars form starches.	Primarily found in grains (rice, wheat, or cornmeal and *masa harina*), and vegetables (potatoes and plantains).
Glycogen	The starch in the body that stores sugars.	Found in the liver and muscles.
Dietary fiber	Carbohydrates that are not digestible by humans but have other important functions.	Primarily found in the outer covering of grains (e.g., Whole wheat, or the "bran"), and in vegetables and fruits.

Proteins

Proteins are called the building blocks of life. They build or repair tissue. Our heart, skin, muscles, blood, nails, and the antibodies that help us fight off diseases contain proteins. EVERY part of our body has some or is almost all protein! Protein is made up of different combinations of amino acids.

Essential Amino Acids

There are about 20 amino acids that are important to human nutrition, but nine of them are considered *essential*. They are essential because the body cannot make these amino acids, and so it must get them through the foods we eat.

Imagine that the disease protection factor in our body is a sign that says "STOP." To make a STOP you need each of the four letters, S, T, O, and P. But you only have the letters S, T, and P. You need to get the letter or the materials to make the letter O. Until you do, you will not be able to make the protective factor STOP. Likewise, to make a protein, we need the necessary amino acids in the correct amounts.

So, it is important to:

1. *Eat foods that supply your body with all the essential amino acids.* Meats, fish, poultry, milk, eggs, and cheese have all the essential amino acids in adequate amounts, so they are considered *complete proteins*, **or**

2. *Combine or eat the right "incomplete protein" foods* to get all the essential amino acids that you need, and in the right amounts. Grains and beans (such as tortillas and beans, or rice and beans) are a common combination of complementary proteins.

Complementary Proteins

Foods that have some but not all the essential amino acids or the adequate amounts are *still important sources* of proteins. But be sure that, over time, you are eating the right combinations, so that you are getting all the amino acids you need. This is VERY important, especially for **vegetarians.**

Complementary Proteins—Combination Ideas		
Complete and Incomplete Protein Combinations		
Complete Protein	Incomplete Protein	**Example of Foods Or Dishes**
Milk	Grains	Milk and rice soup, rice pudding
Cheese	Grains	Macaroni and cheese, *arepas* with cheese, pizza
Meat or fish	Grains	Rice with chicken or codfish
Eggs	Grains	Eggs in a corn or flour tortilla
Incomplete Protein Combinations That Form Complete Proteins		
Incomplete Protein	Incomplete Protein	**Examples of Foods Or Dishes**
Legumes	Grains	Rice and beans, tortilla and beans, peanut butter sandwich
Legumes and Seeds	Grains	Hummus (a dip made with garbanzos, sesame seeds, lemon juice, olive oil, and garlic) served with tortillas.
Nuts and Seeds	Grains	A snack of sunflower seeds, peanuts, and crackers

One great way that we can **save money** and **eat nutritionally** is to combine:

a. A small amount of a complete protein (such as meat or fish, which are generally expensive), *and* an incomplete protein (such as rice, bread, or pasta, which are less expensive)

b. *Two or more* incomplete proteins (such as rice and beans, or tortilla and beans)

Popular Dish Combinations That Provide Complete Proteins
a. Hot or cold cereal with milk
b. Meat or cheese pies
c. Cheese sandwiches
d. Tortillas with cheese
e. Rice made with a small amount (pieces) of chicken, meat, or fish
f. Lots of beans with rice (no additional meat with the meal)
g. Plantain pie with cheese and/or meat filling
h. Soup made with vegetables, rice or pasta, and small pieces of chicken, meat, or fish

Fats

Are you confused about fats? Fats are one of the most confusing nutrition topics. There are many different types of fats, their functions are many, and we are constantly hearing about their "good" or "bad" qualities. Let's discuss some basic facts about fats, what they do, the different types and sources.

Functions of fats in foods

In foods, fats provide distinct flavors or odors (think of butter and olive oil). They tenderize (soften) foods; they carry the fat soluble vitamins; and give a soft creamy texture to foods. When used for cooking, some fats produce crispy textures (as in French Fries).

Functions of fats in the body

Fats provide energy (calories) and store energy. Fat cushions and protects many of our organs. The fat under our skin helps us insulate our body and protect it from extreme temperatures. Fats help carry some vitamins (the "fat soluble" or the ones that dissolve in fats) into and throughout our body. Some fats form part of our hormones and other important chemicals or substances in our body.

Some fats are considered essential because they cannot be made by the body. These essential fatty acids are part of hormones, or play an important part of formation of brain and nerve tissues. However, too much fat in the body (especially the saturated fats) and cholesterol, will place us at risk for heart disease.

Sources and Types of Fats: Lipids and Fatty Acids

The scientific word for fat is *lipid*. Basically, fat is a substance that does not dissolve in water. Generally fats are made up of glycerol and three fatty acids, and they are called triglycerides. These fatty acids may be monounsaturated, polyunsaturated, saturated, an omega-3 fatty acid, or a trans fatty acid. We should try to eat mostly the unsaturated types of fats.

Saturation refers to the chemical structure of the fat. The saturated fats tend to be solid at room temperature (like butter), and the unsaturated fats tend to be liquid at room temperature (like olive oil).

If we make liquid fat (that is unsaturated) into a solid, we have added hydrogen and saturated the fat. This will also produce a trans fatty acid. This is the process used to make most margarines and hydrogenated fats (i.e., Crisco®), which are popular for frying and baking.

Each fat is unique in that it contains its own combination of fatty acids. A simple way to illustrate each fat is as follows:

c. Olive oil is primarily made up of *monounsaturated* fatty acids.

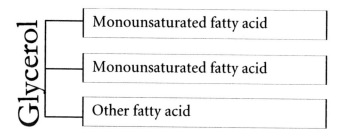

d. Sunflower, safflower, soybean, and corn oils are primarily made up of *polyunsaturated* fatty acids

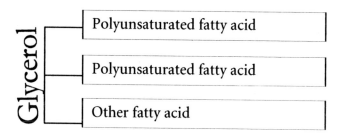

e. Tuna, mackerel, salmon are rich in the highly polyunsaturated *omega-3* fatty acids.

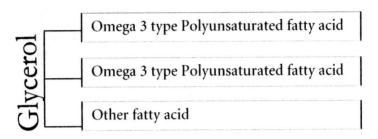

f. Coconut oil and palm oil are primarily made up of *saturated* fatty acids.

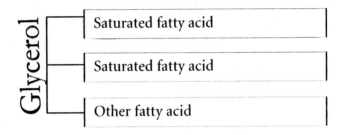

g. Hydrogenated fats and margarines contain *trans* fatty acids.

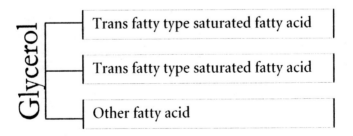

By January 2006 food manufacturers will have to list trans fatty acids, or trans fat, on the Nutrition Facts panel of foods and some dietary supplements.

Sources and Types of Fats: Cholesterol

Cholesterol is a fat-like substance that is found only in foods of animal origin, like butter, lard, meat, fish, poultry, milk, and cheese. Cholesterol in foods is called dietary cholesterol and cholesterol in the blood is called blood or serum cholesterol. Our body also makes its own cholesterol.

Using Calories (Energy) Efficiently

Many Latinos/Hispanics in the U.S. are increasing their intake of fats and sugars. But starches and fiber should make up the major part of our diet and be our major source of energy. Starches provide a steady flow of energy that is relatively inexpensive and easy to digest and use.

If we do not eat enough carbohydrates, our body will use the protein that we eat, or the protein that is stored in our muscles to provide our body with the energy that is needed. Because the primary function of protein is to make or repair tissue, if we do not eat enough carbohydrates during the day, our body will have to use the stored protein for energy.

Usually the foods that provide us with protein like meat and fish are also the most expensive items in our food budget. If we are buying meat and the **meat protein** is being used for energy instead of building tissues, this is very inefficient from a physiological and economic perspective. We could have spent much less money by purchasing bread and had a more efficient source of energy! Therefore, remember to eat enough carbohydrates daily.

Balancing the Calorie Nutrients

So, how do we know how much of each energy nutrient to eat? An easy to remember general guide is:

1. Primarily eat complex carbohydrates (such as the starches from grains and vegetables, not sugars), fruits and other vegetables.

2. Eat a small amount of high quality protein foods, such as chicken or lean meat.

3. Use oil as a small and occasional "accent" item.

The general recommendation is that carbohydrates should be 60% or more of total calories, fats should be less than 30% of total calories, and the remaining calories should come from protein. So, in calorie terms, if you need 2000 calories:

1. 1200 calories should be from carbohydrates (300 grams).

2. 600 or fewer calories should be from fats (65 grams).

3. 200 calories should be from proteins (50 grams).

But an easier guide is to simply remember that the starches in foods like rice, yuca, or potatoes or other grains or vegetables should take up about 2/5 to 3/5 of your plate. Other vegetables should take up about 1/5 to 2/5 of the plate. Meat or meat substitutes should just take up 1/5 of your plate. Fat is just the accent food. This means that, in a **moderate sized plate**, the complex carbohydrates, such as the rice or starchy vegetables, are the main components of the plate. The next items should be your vegetables, and then the milk and meat or their substitutes. The fat, if any, might be the small amount of olive oil that was added to the meat or vegetables.

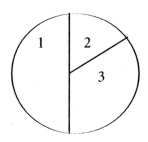

1= Rice, yuca or plantains, etc.
2= Low fat dairy or meat or meat substitutes
3= Other vegetables

CONSUMER TIPS

Carbohydrate Sources

Starches are recommended over sugars for various reasons. Starches are absorbed more slowly (slow absorption is better for controlling insulin and blood sugar levels). They also tend to cause fewer caries (cavities) than simple carbohydrates (sugars). Starches and fiber are usually accompanied by other nutrients. For example, rice, pasta, and bread also have B vitamins, protein and iron, which are not present in sugar. In general, the more refined (processed) a food is, the less fiber and other nutrients it will contain.

Select carbohydrates in the following order:

1. Starches that are also high in fiber (eat very often): such as whole wheat breads, brown rice, oatmeal, bran, whole wheat bagels, bran muffins, green plantains, green bananas, yams, yuca.

2. Combination of starches, fiber, and natural simple sugars (eat often): such as bananas, pears, apples, or other fruits and vegetables.

3. Refined starches (eat occasionally): such as Italian or sliced white breads, enriched white rice, pasta, cornmeal, *masa harina*.

4. Sugars and sugar substitutes (eat less frequently): sugar, honey, sugar alcohols (found in some diet candies), and saccharin.

> **Sugar-free** and **Fat free** *do not mean* **Calorie-free**! Check the food label!

Sugar

Did you know that some of us eat over 150 lbs. of sugar a year? Most of that is consumed in beverages (like colas and coffee), in candies, cakes, or other sweets, or added to foods, like ketchup.

Try to eat less of the added sugar. Get your sugar naturally from fruits and vegetables, where they are accompanied by other nutrients. In addition, the fiber and other constituents in fruits will help absorb the natural sugar more slowly.

> **How many teaspoons of sugar are there in these foods?**
> a. 1 can of cola
> b. 1 tablespoon of catsup
> c. 1 cup of dry sweetened corn cereal flakes
> (**Answers:** a. about 10 tsp.; b. about 1 tsp.; c. 3 tsp.)

Sugar Substitutes

Not all "sweeteners" are carbohydrates. Many people who have diabetes or want to lose weight restrict their sugar intake or use sugar substitutes. These substitutes may or may not provide calories. Each of these products have special properties that must be considered when being used.

Substitute	Information/Uses
Acesulfame potassium	It is about 200 times sweeter than sugar, and provides no calories. This new sugar substitute is used only in some commercial foods. In the U.S. it can be used in candies, tabletop sweeteners, chewing gums, beverages, dessert and dairy product mixes, baked goods, alcoholic beverages, syrups, refrigerated or frozen desserts, and sweet sauces. It can be used in cooking without losing its sweetening power, but does not provide the bulk that sugar provides. It has a slight aftertaste, so it is often mixed with other sweeteners. It is commonly known as Sunette®.
Aspartame	It is about 200 times sweeter than sugar. It is usually found in a blue packet. It provides calories, but we eat very little because of its intense sweetness and thus get few or no calories. Aspartame is used as a tabletop sweetener, in prepared foods, and usually in recipes that do not require long baking or very high temperatures. It breaks down in heat so add it to foods after they have been cooked. It contains phenylalanine, so persons with phenylketonuria (PKU) must be careful about eating foods with aspartame. Common ones are NutraSweet® and Equal®.
Saccharin	It is about 300 times sweeter than sugar, and provides no calories. It is found in a pink packet or in liquid form. It can be used in cooking without losing its sweetening power, and does not provide the bulk or texture that sugar provides. A common one is Sweet 'N Low®
Sucralose	It is 600 times sweeter than sugar and provides no calories. It is made from sugar. In the US it can be used in some low calorie foods, baked goods and mixes, beverages, chewing gum and other foods. and as an over the counter sweetener. It is found in a yellow packet and known as Splenda®.
Sugar alcohols	They contain about the same number of calories as other sugars, but are absorbed by the body more slowly. They include mannitol, sorbitol, and xylitol. Sugar alcohols are generally used in candies and purchased by persons with diabetes. Some people with diabetes may purchase products sweetened with sugar alcohols thinking that they are calorie free. However, this is not the case as they do contain calories.

Protein Sources

Many of the foods that we call "protein foods," such as beef, pork, cheese, eggs and fish, are actually a combination of protein and fat. Others may be a combination of carbohydrates and protein, such as rice, bread, and pasta. Whole milk contains carbohydrate, fat, and protein. Skim milk contains carbohydrates and protein but no fat.

High quality complete protein sources are:

- Lean fish such as cod, trout, or sole
- Canned tuna packed in water
- Lean chicken or turkey without the skin
- Lean meats, such as very lean beef or pork

Fat Sources

It is commonly assumed that our increased intake of fats is, in some part, related to eating out at fast food locations. But, we must also include the fat that we put in foods and the foods that we fry or sauté. In addition, canned meats, canned foods such as spaghetti, or other convenience dishes such as cold cuts or hot dogs are very high in fat. While we may think of these as "protein" foods, we should, in fact, think of them as "fatty" foods or foods with hidden fats and very little protein.

Do you know how much fat is there in these foods?
a. 1 beef hot dog
b. 2 slices salami
c. 1 small package of French Fries
d. 1 slice bacon
e. 1 glass whole milk
f. 1 slice American cheese
(**Answers:** a. 4 tsp., b. 2-1/2 tsp., c. 2-1/2 tsp., d. 1 tsp., e.1-1/2 tsp., f. 2 tsp.)

It's easy to see the "visible" fats, such as butter, margarine, oil, lard, bacon, and cream cheese. But to really control fat intake, you need to be aware of the "hidden or invisible" fats. Common sources of hidden fats include:

- Avocado
- Cake, pie crusts, and other flaky pastries
- Canned meats and many other canned foods
- Cheese
- Chocolates, candies, and mixes such as hot chocolate
- Cookies, croissants, doughnuts, sweet rolls
- Foods with coconut or palm oils
- French fries or fritters
- Ice cream
- Mayonnaise based dishes such as potato and macaroni salads
- Whole and low fat milk
- Nuts
- Olives
- Potato or other chips
- Salad dressings
- Sausages and hot dogs
- Luncheon meats, such as salami, bologna, etc.

ISSUES

The Light and Low Calorie Trap

Despite the increased consumption of low calorie products and fat and sugar substitutes, we are still becoming more overweight. So the general wisdom is that all these products are not really helping us lose weight! Are you caught in this advertising trap, but going nowhere with your weight management goals?

Almost every product has a *light, low calorie, low fat* or *fat free* substitute. With smart choices, this increased availability of options can help us eat healthier foods. However, before you buy that *light, low calorie, low fat* or *fat free* product, ask yourself the following questions:

• Is this product lower in *calories* than its "regular" counterpart?

• Is the serving size (portion) the same as its "regular" counterpart (or smaller)?

• Am I likely to eat the serving size stated, or am I likely to eat more?

• What is the price? Am I willing to pay more for a smaller serving size (portion) or for less fat or sugar?

• Can I buy the "regular item" for a lower price and just eat less?

Carbohydrates—The Misunderstood Calories

Many persons have been told that carbohydrates are high in calories and should be avoided. Potatoes and rice are often called "bad foods" and should be avoided. But we really do need to have some starches in our diet everyday. If there is a problem with carbohydrates, it generally tends to be one of the following two issues:

- We eat *more* carbohydrates than we need and the body turns these extra carbohydrates into fats.
- We eat carbohydrates in combination with a lot of fat (like butter on bread)

For example:

- Portion size—when you eat a piece of Italian bread, how thick do you slice it? A slice the width of your finger is about "right." But many persons I know have a slice that is about the width of their *entire* hand!
- Accompaniments—do you put butter or margarine on bread? If you put a pat of butter on the *small* slice of bread, you are probably getting about 80 calories from the bread and about 45 calories from the butter. In some cases, if you like the butter and spread it on thick, you are probably getting more calories from the butter than from the bread!

Protein—The Misused Calories

Should you be taking amino acid supplements? That is a common question posed to nutritionists, or Registered Dietitians. Most of the time you will hear them respond with "no." This may be a surprise, because protein *is* a very important nutrient. But consider this:

- In the United States and many other developed countries, most people eat more protein than they need;
- Protein sources tend to be one of the most expensive items in a food budget;
- Excess protein is converted to *fat*.

Unless there is a very specific medical reason why a person needs very high amounts of protein, it is generally not advisable to take amino acid supplements, which are *very* expensive. Why tell someone to pay all that money to get fat? More protein will not build more muscle. More muscle is built with specific toning exercises and a good muscle training program.

Fat—The Over Consumed Food

Why is there such an emphasis on eating less fat? Because most persons obtain more than one third of their calories through fats. It is recommended that our diet contain 30% or fewer calories from fats.

But eating less fats is very difficult, especially if we eat out, or are in a hurry. Fried foods are quick to make, are available just about everywhere, and tend to be less costly than non-fried foods. They are also *easy to hold with one hand* (so we can drive!).

How can we avoid consuming more fat when eating out or buying foods in a hurry?

• Ask for the small, plain burger.

• Ask for the grilled chicken or broiled fish sandwich, plain.

• Skip the French Fries, or only have a small portion about once a month.

• Have a salad with the fat free dressing, or a dash of your favorite flavored vinegar or lemon juice.

• Have fruit such as apples, bananas, or grapes as a snack.

Some eateries have calorie cards. Get one, carry it around, and use it to make appropriate food choices.

CONTEMPORARY LATINO/HISPANIC LIFE

Carbohydrates and Preventing Caries (Cavities)

Well cared for teeth are beautiful. In contemporary society, prevention of caries (decay and deterioration of dental enamel) is the area of emphasis in dental care. Caries are caused when carbohydrates are converted to acid by bacteria in the mouth. The following conditions promote this activity:

- **Type of foods**: high carbohydrate foods, especially sugars, are converted to acids

- **Length of time the food is in the mouth**: the longer the food is in the mouth, the more time it has to be converted to acid

- **Stickiness of the food:** the stickier the food, the more it clings to the teeth and promotes acid production

Common Caries Creating Scenarios:	Possible Solutions:
Sipping coffee with milk and sugar while working at your desk.	Drink the coffee at one time, during a break, then sip water to cleanse the mouth.
Sipping soda while at the beach.	Sip water throughout the day.
Feeding a child sticky foods such as raisins for a snack.	Give raisins and follow up with an apple or water to remove some of the food that has stuck to the teeth.
Eating a sticky candy while out on the road and not brushing your teeth.	Select a less sticky candy, then drink some water.

Favorite Foods to Emphasize

There are many excellent traditional and new foods that Latinos/Hispanics can continue, or start to eat. Corn tortillas, rice, plantains, *yuca*, sweet potatoes, oatmeal, and corn-based cereals are carbohydrate rich sources that provide other nutrients. You can combine these items with traditional lean meats such as turkey or chicken, lean beef or pork, or surimi (imitation crabmeat) or soy based imitation meat products like imitation beef soy granules.

Menu Idea and Preparation Tips	
Menu	Preparation Tips
• **Spanish Omelet Topped with Salsa and Grated Parmesan Cheese** • **Refried Beans** • **Tossed Green Salad** • **Corn Tortillas** • **Orange Spritzer**	• Use egg substitute • Microwave then slice the potatoes • Use non-stick pan and fat free spray • Purchase commercial "fresh" salsa • Purchase canned fat free refried beans
	• Purchase a pre-prepared salad with dark greens and serve with low calorie or calorie free dressing
	• Purchase tortillas • Wrap tortillas in plastic wrap and heat in microwave
	• Mix 8 ounces orange juice with 4 ounces diet ginger ale

There are also many traditional dishes that are very nutritious and good sources of proteins and/or carbohydrates. Some of these, with a few modifications, can easily be made even more nutritious. Here are a few menu ideas:

High Protein Dishes:

- Baked codfish
- Stewed codfish
- Grilled tuna
- Ceviche
- Snapper a la Veracruz
- Marinated Fish

Complex Carbohydrate (starchy) Dishes:

- Pumpkin stew or soup
- Root-vegetable stew
- Pea, lentil, or chickpea stew
- Black bean soup
- Chicken noodle soup
- Stew with starchy vegetables
- Vegetarian "Lasagna" made with pasta, or boiled and mashed ripe plantains and your favorite vegetables.

High Quality Protein and Carbohydrate Combination Desserts:

- Mexican sweet bread with Mexican hot chocolate
- Rice pudding
- Bread pudding
- "Diplomat" Pudding
- *Flan* (made with undiluted low-fat evaporated milk)

Food and Nutrition in This Millennium

Future food trends and nutrition guidelines may focus on the following:

- The percent (or amount) of carbohydrates, proteins, and fat calories that should make up our diet. But complex carbohydrates will continue to be the best, safest, and most economical source of calories.

- More use of different grains, such as amaranth, quinoa, flavored and different shaped pastas, flavored rices, along with starchy vegetables such as potatoes, *yuca*, and sweet potato.

- The "best" fats or the "best" amounts for persons with specific disease conditions, such as cancer or heart disease. There will be even more emphasis on how to eat to prevent getting these diseases.

- Alternatives to meat, especially beef. This will include lean meats such as pork loin and non-traditional meats such as ostrich or rabbit, and non-meats such as textured vegetable proteins and plant based meat substitutes like vegetarian hamburger patties.

- Continued use of existing and new fat and sugar substitutes. There will be more information on the dangers and risks concerning their use, and the setting of "safe" and/or "dangerous" levels.

Chapter 4
Vitamins and Minerals

The Difference Between Vitamins and Minerals

Do you give your children vitamin or mineral pills because they are "good for them?" Perhaps you remember being given cod fish liver oil because it was good for you. Many of us take these pills or supplements even if we do not know how they work. We need to know about these nutrients to make wise decisions about what foods to eat, whether or not to take additional vitamins and minerals, and the amounts to take.

Vitamins

Definition. Vitamins do not provide calories, but they work with other compounds to perform a variety of functions. This can range from protecting the skin, to helping the body fight a cold. Vitamins are important regulators of many body functions. Some vitamins need other substances to be absorbed or used, or help absorb or use other nutrients.

Vitamins are needed in small amounts and that is why they are called micronutrients. But they should not be forgotten or ignored just because they are needed in small amounts. The lack of a vitamin will cause a specific deficiency, so there are recommended intakes for vitamins. These recommended amounts meet the needs of most healthy people.

Types. There are two categories of vitamins; the water-soluble (dissolved in water) and the fat soluble (dissolved in fat).

Water-Soluble Vitamins. The water-soluble vitamins include vitamin C (ascorbic acid) and the B complex vitamins, which are thiamin, riboflavin, niacin, folate, vitamin B12, vitamin B6, biotin, and pantothenic acid. Thiamin, riboflavin, niacin, biotin, and pantothenic acid are important in energy (calorie) metabolism. Folate and vitamin B12 help make new cells. Vitamin B6 helps make hemoglobin (which carries oxygen in the blood) and proteins. Vitamin C helps prevent oxidation and helps form the "glue" needed by cells (such as for healing). Vitamin C is also a part of the immune response (it helps the body protect itself against infections).

Every vitamin has many functions, and some of these functions may require more than one nutrient. For example, to use calories (energy) you need at least five nutrients. So it is important not to assume that the "tiredness" one feels is from a deficiency of one specific vitamin. The cause can be one or more nutrients, or just lack of sleep. Because water-soluble vitamins dissolve in water, foods rich in these nutrients should not be cooked in large amounts of water.

Some Sources of Water Soluble Vitamins	
Vitamin	Sources
Thiamin	Pork, ham, liver, whole grains, beans, nuts
Riboflavin	Milk, yogurt, cottage cheese, meat, leafy green vegetables, whole grains, enriched breads, and cereals
Niacin	Milk, eggs, meat, poultry, fish, whole grains, enriched breads and cereals, nuts
Folate	Leafy green vegetables, beans, seeds, liver
Vitamin B12	All animal foods (meats, milk, cheese, eggs, fish, etc.)
Vitamin B6	Green and leafy vegetables, meats, fish, poultry, shellfish, beans, fruits, whole grains
Biotin	Found in all foods
Pantothenic acid	Found in almost all foods
Vitamin C	Citrus fruits, pineapple, melon, cabbage, dark green vegetables, cantaloupe, strawberries, peppers, tomatoes, potatoes, mango, papaya

Fat Soluble Vitamins. The fat soluble vitamins are A, D, E, and K. Like the water-soluble vitamins, every fat soluble vitamin has many functions. Vitamin A is best known for its role in helping prevent night blindness. But Vitamin A is also important in maintaining healthy skin and tissues as well as defending against infections. Vitamin D is important for making some hormones and in regulating the levels of calcium in the blood. With the help of sunlight, the body can also make vitamin D. Vitamin E is an antioxidant and is important in maintaining fat storage, and vitamin K is important in blood clotting.

The fat soluble vitamins dissolve in fat, and so they are not "lost" in water when cooking. In the body, the fat soluble vitamins are "tied" to a protein molecule so they can be carried throughout the body. These are called lipoproteins. Fat soluble vitamins are stored in tissues, so high amounts may be toxic. So, it is important to obtain enough of these vitamins through foods and not use supplements that may provide excessively high or dangerous amounts.

Some Sources of Fat Soluble Vitamins	
Vitamin	**Sources**
A	Dark orange fruits and vegetables such as mango, papaya, and sweet potato; spinach and other dark leafy green vegetables, such as broccoli; fortified milk and cheese.
D	Fortified milk, margarine, eggs, liver, sardines. Sunlight on the skin also helps the body make vitamin D.
E	Polyunsaturated fats and oils, green leafy vegetables, wheat germ, whole grains, nuts, seeds.
K	Liver, green leafy vegetables, cabbage, milk. Some bacteria can make it in the intestinal tract.

Minerals

Definition. When you hear the word mineral, you may think only of rocks, but the body also requires some of these inorganic elements. Minerals, like vitamins, do not provide calories, but they are important in helping the body perform a variety of functions. For example, calcium helps make up our bones, it helps with blood clotting, and with muscle contractions.

Types. There are two classifications of the minerals. There are the major minerals (macrominerals) and the trace minerals (microminerals). The major minerals include calcium, chloride, magnesium, phosphorus, potassium, sodium, and sulfur. The trace minerals include iron, zinc, iodine, selenium, copper, manganese, fluoride, chromium, cobalt, and molybdenum. It is also suspected that we need several other minerals such as nickel, silicon, and boron. But we do not know enough about these minerals yet to say that they are definitely needed by humans.

The Major Minerals (Macrominerals).

1. Calcium is important in bone structure, the regulation of muscle contractions, blood clotting, and nerve impulses.

2. Chloride helps maintain fluid balance and it is part of the hydrochloric acid in the stomach, which is important for digestion.

3. Magnesium is important in energy reactions, muscle contractions, and blood clotting.

4. Phosphorus is also part of bone structure and it is necessary for growth and energy reactions.

5. Potassium is important in maintaining fluid balance inside the cells.

6. Sodium helps regulate the fluids around the cells and fluids that circulate throughout the body.

7. Sulfur is a part of many proteins.

Trace Minerals (Microminerals).

Although trace minerals are needed in very small amounts (together they probably would not fill a teaspoon) they have very important functions in the body.

1. Iron is an important carrier of oxygen in the blood and in muscles.
2. Zinc is an important part of both the muscles and taste perception, and it is part of many enzymes.
3. Iodine is important in regulating body temperature and metabolism, reproduction, blood cell production, and many other functions.
4. Selenium and copper have important antioxidant properties.
5. Manganese is important in metabolism.
6. Fluoride is important in the structure of bones and teeth.

CONSUMER TIPS

DRI's, RDA's, AI's, DV's: What Do They Mean?

How much of a vitamin or mineral a person needs is a complicated matter. The needs are related to age, gender, health status, lifestyle and other specific individual needs. In the U.S., there are various terms and guidelines that are used related to needs and intakes of various nutrients.

The Dietary Reference Intake (DRI) is a general term that refers to the various recommendations, but in general DRI is used to mean the daily nutrient recommendations. These are based on age and sex. The DRI include the Recommended Dietary Allowances (RDAs) and the Adequate Intakes (AI). The DVs are the Daily Values. These are the reference requirements used on the food labels. The RDA's are the amounts recommended for specific ages and genders. The AI are general guidelines for nutrients for which we do not know enough about, and have not determined a specific amounts or need for different age groups or genders.

Sodium—A Potentially Harmful Nutrient

Do you know someone who has high blood pressure and has been told not to eat a lot of salt? Well, this person is eating less salt to avoid sodium, a mineral in salt, because chemically, table salt is *sodium* chloride. But table salt is not the only item that should be avoided. Many foods contain natural sodium and processed foods have added sodium.

Why are sodium, salt, or other sodium containing chemicals added to foods? Sodium has many functions in food. Many persons or companies add sodium to foods because it is a very good preservative and helps keep many types of germs from growing on food. Sodium also gives food a unique flavor. Imagine eating eggs, pork chops, or some of your favorite dishes without added salt. Even some sweet foods are high in sodium.

As a result of eating processed foods, we take in more sodium than we need. For example, consider that regular oatmeal has about 2 mg. of sodium. But instant oatmeal, a more processed product, has about 283 mg. of sodium. Imagine eating five or six processed items a day. But as we get used to the flavor and high level of salt in these foods, we want and eat even more salt.

It is very important to read food labels to know the amount of sodium in food. The food label has information about the amount of sodium in the food per serving. The list of ingredients may also say monosodium glutamate, sodium phosphate, sodium nitrate, or have other terms with the word "sodium." This means that the food has added sodium.

Sodium Terms on U.S. Food Labels
Sodium Free—Less than 5 mg. per serving
Very Low Sodium—35 mg. or less per serving
Low Sodium—140 mg. or less per serving

Even foods made at home will be very high in sodium if we use commercial seasonings such as *adobos or moles, or commercial salsas* and salt to season our food. For us, the more natural or unsalted foods taste bland, so we also add salt to foods at the table. Do you know someone who adds salt to food without even tasting it first? Even our children, who are growing up used to many instant and canned foods, cold cuts, and salty snacks are adding more salt to their diets. That is why most of us are eating much more sodium than we really need. Try to eat mostly fresh and less processed foods.

ISSUES

Vitamin And Mineral Supplements

The easy availability of pills or supplements can be one of the advantages and disadvantages of living in a modern society, so we need to be careful not to abuse these products. Vitamin and mineral supplements are discussed in chapter 6, Dietary Supplements and Other Products.

Is Any Amount Safe?

When deciding how much of a vitamin or mineral is needed, several things are considered. This includes the amount needed to prevent the deficiency disease, the range or amount needed to be healthy, and the levels that may be either too much or harmful. So, for example, when purchasing a vitamin pill, it is important to read the label and find out how much you are getting from the pill. The label will tell you whether you are getting 50%, 100%, 150%, or more of the recommended amounts. Remember that in addition to what you are getting through the pill, you will also get some of the nutrient through your foods.

What Is A *Megadose*?

A *high potency* product has 100 percent or more of the Daily Value. A dose that is ten or more times more than the recommended amount is considered a *megadose*, and generally not recommended. Think of it this way. Would you eat ten times more calories than you need? What would be the results?

It seems that some vitamins, including the water soluble ones, (such as the B vitamins or vitamin C) can create health problems if taken in large amounts. Fat soluble vitamins (such as vitamin A) can accumulate in the body's fat and be harmful if taken in large amounts over a long period of time.

Quick Ways to Add Calcium and Iron to Your Diet
Calcium
<ul><li>Top your favorite dishes with shredded, low fat cheese.</li><li>Add 1/2 cup powdered dry skim milk to 1 quart of fluid skim milk.</li><li>Use undiluted evaporated skim milk in recipes that call for regular milk or cream.</li></ul>
Iron
<ul><li>Cook foods in an iron skillet.</li><li>Add small pieces of lean meat to bean dishes.</li><li>Drink orange, grapefruit, or pineapple juice with breads, grains, or vegetable dishes.</li></ul>

Non Vitamins

You may hear some claims that the following are also vitamins: inositol, lipoic acid, choline, B15 (pangamic acid) and vitamin B17 (laetrile). As a consumer, it is important for you to know that technically, these are not vitamins. Pangamic acid has been primarily marketed to athletes, and laetrile has been marketed to persons with cancer. The claims for these chemicals have not been proven. In some cases, some of these compounds, as purchased or used, may even be dangerous.

CONTEMPORARY LATINO/HISPANIC LIFE

Are You Too Busy to Eat Well?

Many of us take vitamin or mineral pills because we believe we are too busy to eat well, or do not have time to eat. I have heard this comment from clients. Another comment, which worries me more, is when parents tell me that they give their children a vitamin pill because the child may not have time to eat. While it may be advantageous to give your child a safety margin with a multivitamin and mineral supplement, consider the following:

- A multi vitamin and/or mineral pill *does not* provide the energy (calories) that we need for everyday functioning. Remember, energy is provided through the foods that give us carbohydrates, proteins, and fats.

- A solitary vitamin or mineral (such as vitamin C) will provide *only* that nutrient. We still need to eat well to get all the other nutrients we need.

- Taking a pill may give us a false sense of security that further discourages us from making an effort to eat well.

- What type of message are we sending our children when we tell them to take a vitamin or mineral pill? Do we want to imply that there is an easy way out or that they can "skip" healthy habits?

Favorite Foods to Emphasize

Latino/Hispanic foods include a wide variety of vitamin and mineral sources. Planned well, the common diet provides many vitamins and minerals.

Some Menu Examples	
Meals	
Example 1	Hot oatmeal made with skim milk Orange juice Whole wheat roll or tortilla Hot chocolate made with skim milk
Example 2	Cuban sandwich Watercress salad *Mamey* fruit shake
Example 3	Red beans and rice Baked ripe plantain Tossed salad Pineapple juice
Example 4	Green peppers stuffed with rice and ground beef Tossed dark greens with tomato wedges and Spanish onion Fresh lemonade

Snacks and Desserts	
Example 1	Tropical fruit salad Pineapple or pumpkin *Flan* Frozen mango dessert (ice milk and mango puree)

Food and Nutrition in This Millennium

In the past, we considered vitamins important because of their role in disease prevention. That will continue to be important, especially in areas where, for a variety of reasons, there is undernutrition. However, in some areas people will begin or continue to take vitamin and mineral pills to make up for what they think is missing in their diet, or for "extra protection or benefits." This can have either positive or negative results.

Possible Positive and Negative Results of Taking Vitamin and Mineral Pills

Possible Positive Results	Possible Negative Results
• Makes us more aware of how we eat and what we do about our health. • Makes us take a more active role in caring for ourselves.	• Makes us neglect how we eat or care for our health because we think we are "already doing something." • If we take too much of a vitamin and the high amount harms us. • We spend more money than we can afford on these products.

This millennium, not only will it be easier to obtain a great variety of Latino/Hispanic foods, it will also be easy to obtain other ethnic foods that are rich in vitamins and minerals. There will be more emphasis on having all people try and use more of these foods either alone or as "fusion cuisine." Also, there will be new genetically engineered varieties of fruits and vegetables that are even higher in some vitamins and minerals than their traditional varieties. We will have more opportunities to eat combinations of great foods. These will be among the great advantages of this millennium!

Chapter 5
Herbs and Phytochemicals

Introduction

Transportation is making what were difficult-to-find herbs and exotic foods (some which may be new to other persons, but common to us) more popular and available almost any time of the year. A result of an increasing general interest in different herbs and exotic foods also means that these items are now found in supermarkets, not just specialty or ethnic food stores.

Herbs and Spices

Throughout the world, the various parts of a plant, such as the seeds or leaves, may be used for a variety of purposes. Spices grow in tropical areas and are the stems, seeds, roots, fruits, buds, or bark of plants or trees. Herbs grow in temperate climates and are the leaves of plants.

Culinary Uses of Herbs and Spices

From a culinary perspective, herbs and spices are used as garnishes in foods and in cooking. We use aniseed, bay leaves, cumin, coriander (cilantro), oregano, parsley, rosemary, sesame seed, thyme, and many other herbs and spices. The trend is toward their continued use, especially when creating traditional and the new, great, "fusion" cuisine (the mixture of different ethnic foods).

Tips for Using and Caring for Your Culinary Herbs

1. One tablespoon of fresh herb is about 1 to 1 1/2 teaspoons of dried herb.

2. When trying a new herb or spice, add a little first (about 1/4 teaspoon), then more. It's easier to add more than to *remove* too much!

3. Try one new herb at a time on a mild food. Give yourself at least three different "tries" before you decide that you do not like it (for example, dill in a potato salad, dill on chicken, dill in rice). Remember, new tastes are learned and cultivated!

4. Store spices and herbs in a dark, cool, and dry place. Heat, light and air destroy them.

5. Use an ice cube tray to freeze individual herbs in water or make an herb puree. When frozen, remove the cubes and seal them in a plastic freezer bag.

6. Wash and dry herbs and freeze them in a sealed plastic bag.

7. To dry herbs, wash and place them in paper towels and dry them on a low setting in the microwave oven for two or three minutes. Seal tightly and store.

8. To test their freshness, rub them between your fingers. If you do not smell their fragrance, or if they look yellowish or gray, they are old. Throw them out!

9. When using an herb or spice for the first time, use it alone. That way, if someone has an allergic reaction to it, you will know immediately what herb or spice may have caused the reaction.

Create your own fusion cuisine and new family traditions by mixing different herbs and spices with traditional and modern elements, such as boiled yuca with rosemary, or rice pudding topped with anise seed or mint.

The increased availability of herbs and spices is changing what we think about and how we prepare foods. Many herbs and spices are safe to use in moderate amounts and are great in foods. You can then add "new" spices along with "old" ones to your favorite dishes. Sliced tomatoes can be topped with fresh cilantro, oregano, basil, or thyme. It can be a different salad every day of the week!

> • Make gourmet vinegar by adding your favorite herb, such as cilantro or basil!

Medicinal Uses of Herbs and Spices

The use of herbs for medicinal purposes is a part of traditional healing of various cultures, including Latinos. Although herbs or spices may be used as a seasoning ingredient, teas, tisanes, or infusions are also made from herbs and spices, and are used for medicinal purposes. Herbs and spices are used by some persons to treat colds, coughs, fevers, for relaxation, to aid digestion, during childbearing, to treat the eyes and mouth, and as first aid for cuts, wounds, boils, or insect bites.

New scientific information about safe uses and dangers of some herbs has reawakened interest in the medicinal qualities of herbs. For many of us, this new information confirms the wisdom of some traditional practices.

In the U.S., herbs, spices, or foodstuffs that are commonly used for health purposes include chamomile, echinacea, feverfew, foxglove, garlic, ginger, ginkgo biloba, ginseng, goldenseal, kava kava, St. John's Wort, saw palmetto, and valerian. Herbs that appear safe in teas include chamomile and mint.

Almost all herbs have the potential for being dangerous (including the common ones mentioned above), especially if taken in large amounts or if the person is allergic or sensitive to one of their components. Some that are known to be **dangerous** are aconite, belladonna, blue cohosh, borage, broom, chaparral, comfrey, ephedra (ma huang), germander, kombucha tea, lobelia, pennyroyal, poke root, sassafras, scullcap, yohimbe, and others. But even the commonly used herbs, St. John's Wort, gingko biloba, and kava kava, may be harmful.

The common conditions that may make the use of an herb or herb supplement dangerous include taking it in large concentrations and/or for long periods of time, using a poor quality product, or having an allergy to a component in the herb. Occasionally over-the-counter or prescription medications may interact with the herb supplements. You want to be sure that the herb and other medications are a safe combination. Check with your physician before using any herb supplement.

I like to remind persons that ask me about herb supplements that our traditional practices did not encourage consumption of extracted or concentrated versions of these items, or their consumption in very large doses.

Herbal Supplements—How They Are Used		
Supplement	**Used For**	**Comments**
Chamomile	Relieving digestive problems.	There are not enough data to evaluate these claims. Pregnant and breast-feeding women should avoid the use of chamomile **supplements**, as safety data are lacking (occasional tea is probably okay).
Garlic	Boosting immunity, and lowering blood cholesterol levels.	Results evaluating the claim that garlic lowers blood cholesterol are inconclusive as data are conflicting. There are not enough data to evaluate the effectiveness of garlic in boosting immunity. If used, garlic **supplements** should be part of a medically supervised cholesterol lowering program. General use in cooking is okay.
Ginger	Reducing nausea and vomiting.	Results evaluating claims are inconclusive as data are conflicting. Pregnant women should avoid the use of ginger **supplements** as safety data are lacking. General use in cooking is okay.
Gingko	Improving mental alertness, and overall brain function.	There are not enough data to evaluate these claims. Pregnant women should avoid the use of Gingko supplements as safety data are lacking. Avoid giving this **supplement** to children as there is an associated risk of seizures.

Ginseng	Enhancing physical and mental performance.	There are risks associated with the use of ginseng. Persons with diabetes should exercise caution in the use of this supplement. Pregnant and breast-feeding women should avoid the use of the supplements as safety data are lacking.
Kava Kava	Relieving anxiety, stress, and restlessness.	There are not enough data to evaluate these claims. Chronic heavy use of Kava Kava supplements can have adverse effects. Pregnant and breast-feeding women, and children under the age of 12 years should avoid the use of the supplements as safety data are lacking.
Ma Huang (Ephedra)	Suppressing appetite, stimulating the central nervous system, and relieving symptoms in asthma.	Ma Huang has been used for some illnesses under medical supervision but it is dangerous and has been linked to some deaths. **Do not** use Ma Huang without the approval and supervision of a physician. Pregnant women should avoid the use of Ma Huang.
Mint	Aiding digestion, relieving flatulence, and relieving pain.	The ingestion of mint for purposes other than flavoring is not advisable, as safety data are lacking. Occasional tea or general use in cooking is okay.
St. John's Wort	Treating depression.	There is not enough evidence to support the use of St. John's Wort supplements in the use of depression. Pregnant and breast-feeding women and children should avoid the use of St. Johns Wort supplements as safety data are lacking.
Valerian	Sedative purposes.	Pregnant and breast-feeding women, and children should avoid the use of valerian **supplements** as safety data are lacking.

Teas

There are three types of teas: 1) fermented (regular tea), 2) semi-fermented, or 3) green. Regular tea is fermented, that is, the leaves have been oxidized, which causes them to turn brown. Green tea is made using fresh herbs. Some teas have regular (fermented) tea leaves and herbs, others are *herbal teas*, and others are a combination of ingredients, such as tea leaves, herb, flowers, spices, and/or other flavorings. Most teas contain caffeine (yes, even herbal teas). If you want *decaffeinated* tea, purchase caffeine free tea or caffeine free herbal tea.

For some Latinos, teas are a beverage to be consumed when we are ill. But more of us are drinking iced teas as a daily beverage. Flavored teas are increasing in popularity. You can purchase them flavored or create your own. For example, you can grow mint, chamomile or other herbs and make your own green teas. We can also make our own flavored teas. Here are a few ideas for making fancy iced teas:

Ideas for Your Own Flavored Tea
- Add a few drops of lime or lemon juice
- Add a few drops of apple, pineapple, or other juice
- Add an herb or spice such as mint, a cinnamon stick, or anise seed
- Add a drop of flavoring extract, such as orange extract
- Add a flavoring syrup, such as cherry flavor

Phytochemicals

Although phytochemicals are not classified as required nutrients, they are revolutionizing and challenging our traditional ideas about nutrition. The term "phytochemical" will be common in this millennium. Understanding what phytochemicals are will help us make healthy food choices and focus on eating well to *prevent disease.*

"Phyton" means vegetable or plant in Greek. The word "phytochemical" is a general term that refers to many different compounds found in plant foods. Phytochemicals help prevent or aid in the treatment of some of the leading causes of death—cancer, diabetes, cardiovascular disease, and hypertension. Some phytochemicals may have anti-heart disease and anti-cancer properties. Others relieve symptoms associated with menopause such as hot flashes and night sweats.

The number of compounds that are classified as phytochemicals is very long (thousands!). To complicate the issue, the **different** phytochemicals found in **different** fruits and vegetables have **different** protective qualities. This strengthens the argument that one should eat many **different** fruits and vegetables.

Trying to determine what foods to eat in order to get the beneficial effects of phytochemicals is simple. As it turns out, most of the phytochemicals are found in foods that are common in Latino dishes. For example, onions and garlic are used extensively in Hispanic cooking. We add tomatoes, onions, peppers, and garlic to salsas, soups, bean, meat, or rice dishes. We even put some of these foods in salads. Citrus fruits are staple Latino foods. We eat oranges and grapefruits; drink their juice, and use limes and lemons to make beverages or seasonings. These are positive behaviors that should be continued.

Did you know any one fruit and vegetables can have hundreds, or thousands, of phytochemicals? Can you imagine what a food label would look like if the phytochemicals had to be listed? So why would we take a pill that contains just one or a few phytochemicals when we can eat the food, which also tastes better? Some broad categories for the many types of phytochemicals includes:

Some Phytochemicals, Possible Benefits, and Sources			
Phytochemical	Possible Benefits	Sources	Comments
Allium or allyl sulfides	May decrease incidence of stomach and intestinal cancer	Onions, garlic	You can remember the vegetables this way: sulfides smell, like onions and garlic
Carotenoids	May have antioxidant (prevents oxidation or aging) effects	Yellow orange and dark greens	Carotenoids are vitamin A precursors (become vitamin A in the body)
Coumarins	May inhibit tumor growth	Citrus fruit	
Dithiolthionnes	May inhibit tumor growth	Broccoli, cabbage (cruciferous vegetables) brussel sprouts	You can remember these cruciferous vegetables this way: their leaves "cross" each other.
Indoles	May have anticancer properties	Broccoli, cabbage, cauliflower, brussel sprouts	

Isoflavones (phytoestrogens)	May lower blood cholesterol levels and symptoms of menopause.	Soybeans, whole grain cereals	Soybean has high levels of genistein, an isoflavone used as part of natural hormone replacement therapy.
Isothyocyanates and thiocyanates	May inhibit tumors	Broccoli, cabbage, cauliflower	
Limonene	Helps make anticancer compounds (enzymes)	Citrus fruit	Remember: lime, limonene
Phenols and polyphenols	Helps make anticancer compounds (enzymes)	Fruits, vegetables, and green (herbal) tea	
Saponins	May help decrease incidence of colon cancer	Soybeans, other legumes, soy milk	
Sterols (B sitosterol)	May help lower cholesterol	Vegetables and vegetable oils (like olive oil)	

Why We Think They Promote Health

Phytochemicals are a new weapon in disease prevention and treatment. We know that eating a diet high in fruits, vegetables, legumes, nuts, and whole grains seems to protect against heart disease and cancer.

There are various ways this protection is provided. A possible way may be production of chemicals that help block some of the actions related to the development of cancer. Also, some phytochemicals seem to lower blood cholesterol levels or prevent growth of specific cancer cells. Some phytochemicals seem to block oxidation of cells or prevent DNA (cell production) damage. Isoflavones seem to help relieve the symptoms associated with menopause. Phytochemicals may work alone, or along with other chemicals, including vitamins or minerals.

So, try to eat a lot of different and delicious fruits, vegetables, and whole grains (such as oatmeal) as you move toward health promotion!

An easy guide for getting lots of different phytochemicals and benefiting from their various protective functions are to eat:

- garlic, and onions
- citrus fruits and berries,
- different types of beans,
- dark green and yellow fruits and vegetables,
- cabbage, cauliflower, broccoli, dark leafy greens or cruciferous vegetables (vegetables that have leaves that "cross" each other).

!!!!! Hot Chili Pepper !!!!!

Did you know that hot chili peppers contain the phytochemical capsaicin, which may help prevent lung and other cancers? Cilantro has a high anti-cancer activity. Put some chopped cilantro and hot chili peppers in your favorite vinegar and heat up the flavor of your favorite *tostones* (*patacones*) with a dash of your own flavored vinegar!

CONSUMER TIPS

Sources of Phytochemicals

Fruits and vegetables to emphasize include: garlic, grapes, onions, citrus fruits, soybeans and other legumes, strawberries, broccoli, cantaloupe, cauliflower, cabbage, celery, carrots, tomatoes, peppers, cucumber. Cilantro is a good source of phytochemicals.

Remember, one food will contain many different phytochemicals, which will provide, for the money, more flavor and variety than a pill. If you do purchase pills, be a careful consumer. Find out if the company has high packaging standards, if the pill contains safe levels, the side effects, and if the pill has an *active* form of the chemical before you spend your money!

ISSUES

Herbal and Phytochemical Supplements

Among the issues or concerns about the purchase and use of phyto-chemicals are: the lack of regulation of herbs and other types of supplements, and the lack of information about the safety of taking concentrated amounts.

As a result of the interest in phytochemicals, there has also been an increase in over-the-counter pills with specific phytochemicals (such as isoflavone pills). It is still not clear if the pill form of the chemicals is as good as (or better than) the origin of the phytochemical, the food itself. In some cases, the pills do not contain the active form of the chemical that is found in the herb. We also do not know how many, or in what combination these chemicals should be consumed. We do not know how much, if any, of these chemicals we need.

Also, because herbs are called "foods," they are not regulated for safety or effectiveness by the Food and Drug Administration (FDA). So, the pills you are buying may or may not have the active ingredient found in the naturally occurring food, or may not have been processed safely. These items do not have to be tested before they are put in the market. They can only be taken off the market if there is proof that the advertising to sell the product was not truthful, or there is proof that people have been harmed by the product. That enables many of these products to be in the market, but it means that the con-sumer has to careful.

CONTEMPORARY LATINO/HISPANIC LIFE

Phytochemicals exist naturally in fruits, vegetables, and grains. These scientific names, once scary to consumers, have long been known to food scientists. They knew that these compounds had important functional qualities (for example, that some compounds help give foods their odor). But only recently have we discovered that phytochemicals also contain protective substances too. However, there are many questions that still need to be answered about these chemicals.

Why Are Phytochemicals Not Considered Required "Nutrients"?

The traditional definition for a required nutrient is that the compound is not *made* by the body, that its absence will *cause* a specific deficiency disease, and that providing the compound will *eliminate* the deficiency disease. There is usually a set recommended level of intake for the nutrient.

While phytochemicals seem to help prevent some diseases, we have not yet "proven" that their absence causes a disease. In some cases, we know that it does not. For example, as far as we know, it is not the absence of allium that causes stomach cancer.

Are Pills Better Than Foods?

Information about the disease-preventing qualities of phytochemicals is new. We do not know if a single phytochemical is as effective as their combinations. There are many different types of these chemicals in foods. For now, the easy way to get a wide range of these beneficial compounds is through foods. We do not know what amounts are "safe levels" to put into pills. A compound may be available in a small amount in herbal tea. But is the synthetic, concentrated form harmful or (even) more beneficial than that found in the plant?

Likewise, there is an assumption about the "inherited wisdom" concerning the value of herbs, but we do not yet have scientific proof of "cause and effect" for some of these traditional practices. These data are hard to get because there are hundreds of compounds in herbs. For example, how do we know which compound, and in what concentration or form, is effective? This will take many years to determine. So, continue to enjoy your chamomile tea, but drink it in moderate amounts!

Future Trends

This millennium more foods will be fortified or enhanced nutritionally by adding more phytochemicals, or adding some of the chemicals found in herbs. Chosen wisely, these new foods will enable you to enhance the variety and quality of your diet. How can we keep positive habits and use new ones to improve our overall health? Ask yourself:

- How is this product better or worse than the traditional?

- Is it better to take garlic pills instead of continuing to use garlic in cooking?

- Is it better to eat an orange or have a fortified orange-flavored candy?

- Is it better to drink lemon flavored soda or drink homemade limeade?

- If I take a pill with a phytochemical, what is the trade-off (in terms of your health and money)? How am I obtaining other phytochemicals or other nutrients?

A Food From the Past Is the Food of the Future!

If you are not familiar with soybeans, remember that you can purchase and use them as you would your favorite beans. You can drink the vanilla flavored soymilk instead of sodas or colas, or buy the textured vegetable protein (TVP), or soybean granules and use them in place of the ground meat when making *picadillo, pastelon, empanadas,* or chili. This substitution will also decrease the amount of fat in your dish!

Favorite Foods to Consider

The good news is that we already eat foods that contain phytochemicals. What we need to do now is try to **eat more** of them. If we do this and also decrease the amount of meats and saturated fats that we eat, we will have improved the cancer preventing quality of our diet!

Some ideas or suggestions:

Incorporate non-traditional vegetables into traditional mixed dishes.	• In addition to potatoes, add broccoli or other cruciferous vegetables into stews or soups • Use a mixture of dark leafy greens in your salad
Incorporate soy into traditional foods	• Prepare soy beans the way you prepare your favorite black, kidney, or other beans. • Combine textured soy protein flakes or granules with meat in the chili con carne or meat pies or use the soy instead of meat. Soybean products that are delicious include tofu, tempeh, and carob flavored soy milk, which tastes like chocolate milk but is generally lower in sugar, fat, and calories.
Incorporate whole grains into traditional dishes	• Put brown rice instead of white rice into a favorite chicken and rice soup
Increase consumption of green tea	• Serve yourself some hot green tea as an afternoon relaxation snack or when making iced tea, use a mix of half of your favorite tea and half green tea

Many traditional Latino dishes incorporate vegetables. Now the modern market provides fruits and vegetables that were not previously common or available. We can fight cancer and enjoy new culinary adventures by mixing and matching traditional and modern foods.

Food and Nutrition in This Millennium

We already know that some herbs, spices, or phytochemicals in foods have important disease prevention and health related functions. We will continue to hear about discoveries of their benefits and the ways that they help prevent some of the modern day diseases such as cancer and heart disease.

This millennium much of the work will be on identifying the exact functions, benefits, risks, and safe consumption levels of herbs, spices, and phytochemicals. There will probably be recommended intake levels of active ingredients and regulations concerning their processing and sale.

More food products that contain ingredients from herbs or specific phytochemicals will be developed and marketed. If regulations that provide safe production and identify the safe levels that can be added to foods are not developed, as the consumer, you will have to be extra careful to protect yourself and make wise choices at the store. You will see an emphasis on eating a "rainbow diet." This is based on the idea that if you try to eat many different color foods, you will increase your intake of fruits and vegetables, which are low calorie and health promoting foods.

Chapter 6
Dietary Supplements and Other Products

Introduction

Supplements are a big business (billions of dollars annually!). Many of us purchase dietary supplements because we believe that we are at nutritional risk and need these supplements.

In this chapter, I will discuss dietary supplements and products that have been designed for special functions. These supplements include beverages for athletes, pills for persons trying to lose weight, and various kinds of products for persons with special dietary needs.

The United States' Dietary Supplement Health and Education Act has specific definitions for dietary supplements. Products that fall under that definition will be discussed. Products that do not fall within the legal definition of supplements but are often used by us are also discussed here. However, I am discussing these as "formulated products."

Some of these products have common names (such as "sports drinks" such as Gatorade®) but some do not. Therefore, I have also used words that may not be common but will help you categorize or understand the use of certain products. As you read through the book, you will also see that there is an overlapping of categories. For example, we can also call some foods "functional" or "designer" foods.

Hopefully this chapter will help you identify and understand the types of special products that are available, and help you determine which item you need (if any) and how to select it.

United States' Dietary Supplement Health and Education Act

According to the United States' Dietary Supplement Health and Education Act, a **dietary supplement** is a product intended to supplement the diet. It contains a vitamin, mineral, amino acid, herb, or other botanical. A supplement may be a concentrate, metabolite, constituent, extract, or combination of ingredients. Supplements are taken as capsules, powders, softgel, or gelcaps.

The most commonly used supplements are the over-the-counter multivitamin and mineral pills. These supplements can be bought just about anywhere. They can be bought in a supermarket, a community food store such as a *bodega,* or over the Internet. Their easy availability means that more people buy and use these pills.

Types of Supplements

Vitamin and mineral supplements

These products are available as multivitamin and mineral mixes, in combination, or as individual nutrients. You can purchase a "One-A-Day" type multi supplement, a B complex vitamin, or a Vitamin C pill. These supplements are available with doses that range near the 100% RDA values.

Higher doses are also available for some vitamins and minerals. A *high potency* product has more than 100 percent of the RDA. Many of these high potency products are mega doses because they contain more than ten times the RDA. Those pills, taken over long periods of time, may be harmful. This is especially important for the fat soluble vitamins, which are stored in the body.

You should not take high potency pills or megadoses unless there is a specific medical reason, and not without a doctor's supervision. Generally a multivitamin that provides about 100% and not much more of some key nutrients is sufficient. The most common mineral supplements are calcium and iron pills.

Calcium Supplements. There are three important points to consider when buying calcium supplements. First, some calcium supplements are better absorbed than others. Secondly, calcium in a pill is bound to another chemical, so you want to know how much actual (elemental) calcium you are getting from the pill. Thirdly, you need to watch out for potential problems or complications.

In terms of calcium absorption, calcium citrate seems to be the best absorbed. Calcium malate and calcium phosphate dibasic are also well absorbed. The calcium in dolomite (calcium magnesium carbonate), oyster shell, bone meal, or powdered bone are not as well absorbed. Some of these products may even contain harmful materials such as lead.

You can find out how much calcium you are getting from the label. Look for the amount of *elemental calcium*. For example, a product may be 1000 mg. of calcium gluconate, but only 90 mg. of elemental calcium. If you wanted to take in 1000 mg. of calcium through these pills, you would have to take 11 or 12 pills a day. One glass of skim milk is about 300 mg. of calcium. Compare the cost of about 3-1/3 glasses of milk, which would give you about the same amount of calcium to the price of 11 pills. So, purchase pills that have a high amount of elemental calcium.

Be careful about antacids with aluminum or magnesium hydroxide. They may cause calcium loss. Too much calcium may interfere with the absorption of other minerals, especially zinc. If you are taking tetracycline, be careful about calcium and drug interactions. A side effect of some calcium supplements, especially calcium carbonate, is constipation, bloating, and gas.

Iron Supplements. Iron supplements are regularly recommended for infants, children, and women of childbearing age. Purchase your iron supplements in the ferrous form, which is better absorbed than other forms of iron.

Absorption of iron from food sources is increased by vitamin C. So it is recommended that an iron pill be taken with orange juice. Other ways to maximize iron intake include adding a little meat to plant sources, such as pieces of meat in your cooked beans or greens, cooking in iron pots, and not drinking your milk, coffee or tea (which inhibit iron absorption) with the iron rich foods.

Weight loss pills

This is another commonly purchased over-the-counter pill and the components may vary. Many contain PPA (phenylpropanolamine), benzocaine, caffeine or fiber. PPA and caffeine may increase blood pressure. The caffeine stimulates water loss. The benzocaine will reduce the taste or desire for food by numbing the taste buds. Caffeine will stimulate water loss. Pills containing fiber will make one feel full. Some pills contain vitamins and minerals.

Herbal, phytochemical, and other preparations

Herbs pills are popular modern forms of traditional herbs and other products used by many different cultures. Most of these items are safe when used infrequently in a mild tea or infusion. But there is a difference between drinking an occasional cup of herb tea, and taking herb pills everyday.

We are finding that some of these previously assumed safe products, which are now available in concentrated forms, may be harmful if taken over long periods of time or in high concentrations. Some of these may interact with medications or cause allergic reactions. This includes herbal products such as bee pollen, chaparral, comfrey, echinacea, ephedra, feverfew, ginseng, gingko biloba, Jim bu huan, Kombucha tea, and lobelia.

Bodybuilding powders

Muscle or bodybuilding products are popular "powders." Body building products generally contain a mixture of amino acids and/or carbohydrates as their key ingredients. Persons participating in muscle building programs often feel that their training demands that they take amino acids to build muscle. But building muscle is dependent on sufficient total nutrients and spot training.

Some athletes who want to build muscle and boost energy take creatine monohydrate. At certain levels, creatine supplements do seem to help with improved performance during some specific types of physical activity and body muscle. But it is not necessary to purchase supplements, as creatine is found in foods, especially meat and poultry.

Weight loss products

Weight loss beverages or powders have become very popular, in part, from aggressive advertising campaigns. Often these drinks are promoted as a substitute for one or two of the day's meals. They generally have milk or a milk product base, some flavoring, and additional vitamins and nutrients (it's almost like taking a vitamin and mineral pill with a glass of skim milk). These are added to replace some of the nutrients that are probably missing from having the drink instead of a balanced meal.

Nutritional supplements

Another type of supplement that is increasing in popularity (probably from the increased advertising, more than actual need) is the high nutrient drink. These products are especially promoted (but not limited) to persons in specific age groups, such as children or the elderly. Like the weight loss products, I often think of these as little more than a flavored glass of milk with a vitamin/mineral multi supplement. However, persons at a high risk for a nutritional deficiency may very well benefit from these supplements. But, a healthy person probably does not need special supplements merely because he or she is in a particular age group.

Formulated products

I am calling the items listed below formulated products because they do not fall into the dietary supplement category, but may be promoted for special situations or conditions.

Sports Drinks. Sports drinks are not just sold to athletes. These have become common beverages of choice for many people. Most of these drinks contain carbohydrates, sodium, potassium, and other minerals. The carbohydrate will usually be glucose or a form of sugar that is more slowly absorbed. However, in most cases, water alone is sufficient before, during, and after physical activity.

Milk Replacers or Substitutes. There are now many beverages that can be used in place of, or in addition to, milk. These may be grain-based, such as rice drinks, or soy based, such as soymilk. The beverages are available plain or flavored. Vegetarians that avoid dairy products or person that have allergies to milk can use these beverages. If you are using these products instead of milk, check the calcium content. It may be necessary to eat or supplement the diet with other high calcium foods to meet your daily calcium needs.

Breakfast Drinks. Breakfast drinks are often used as a meal substitute and are not much different from nutritional supplement or weight loss drinks.

CONSUMER TIPS

Many contemporary Latinos/Hispanics buy, take, and perhaps depend on vitamin and mineral supplements. The most important thing to remember, as a consumer, is that although there is a law that defines what *can be called a supplement*, these products are not as well regulated as medicines are.

Therefore, these products do not have to be tested and proven safe before they are put on the market. It will be up to you to find out if and how that product may be harmful and if you want to take it. Make sure that you know what you want and that you are purchasing the correct product. If you buy any of these products, get them from a reputable company that has high standards of service, cleanliness, and purity in preparation and packaging.

Does the Function Justify the Price?

Some of these products must be purchased because they are not easily made at home or available. One example is the amino acid product. Amino acids are found in foods, but one cannot find "pure" amino acids. That is another reason why these products tend to be very expensive. A dietary approach may be to try to eat a lot of lean fish or to make some scrambled eggs from egg whites.

Remember, too, that if you take in more amino acids (or proteins) than your body needs, you will convert the extra protein to fat. This also makes the kidneys (and body) work hard, because they must get rid of the extra nitrogen that comes from the amino acids. It is important to read and be familiar with the warnings concerning these products' use.

Can I Make It Myself?

You can make almost an equivalent of some of these items, such as breakfast and sports drinks at home. One could, for example, take a glass of skim milk and add ingredients such as additional powdered dry skim milk, strawberry syrup, and sugar. If you are already taking a vitamin/mineral multi supplement (pill), take it with your homemade drink. Think of it as your own instant breakfast! One can also make a homemade version of a sports drink by mixing about 1 cup juice, 3-4 cups water, and a third teaspoon of salt. Give it a fancy name and share it with your friends!

ISSUES

Among the issues or concerns are: the lack of regulation of herbs and other types of supplements, and the lack of information about the safety of taking concentrated amounts.

Possible Dangers of Some Products

The biggest dangers concerned with the use of these products are the "more is better" myth or their use as "crutch." Consider their benefit versus their risk when deciding whether or not to use them. Remember that they are designed to be *supplements*, not substitutes, to healthy eating.

Vitamin/Mineral or Individual Supplements

Excessive use of the vitamin/mineral supplements may be toxic. This is an especially important concern for children. For example, a cause of some toddlers' deaths is accidental poisoning from iron supplements intended for adults. Also, excessive use of one item (such as vitamin C) may affect the absorption of other vitamins and/or minerals.

Herbal Preparations

The safety or safe levels for herbal preparations are not established. Some herbs do not seem to be dangerous, however some, such as *foxglove,* are very dangerous. Even generally assumed safe herbs may be harmful to specific individuals, as in allergic reactions.

Weight Loss Drinks

Weight loss drinks may be dangerous if the total caloric intake is too low or the protein intake is too high.

Breakfast Drinks

Because many breakfast drinks have a lot of milk or milk products, they are high in lactose. Persons that are lactose intolerant will need to monitor their use of the breakfast (and other) milk based supplements to minimize potential symptoms of lactose intolerance.

CONTEMPORARY LATINO/HISPANIC LIFE

For contemporary Latinos/Hispanics, our ability to function well in modern society will, in large part, be determined by whether or not we can sort out all the information and products available. We need to be able to make choices that apply to our personal life and values. A healthy view of dietary supplements and other foods is to consider them as an "extra" benefit that is available for occasional use and under special circumstances or needs. In reality, we should be in control of their use. These products (like anything else) should not be dominating or overwhelming our life.

What May Be Special Circumstances or Needs?

At certain times we may find that these products have a beneficial function. For example, perhaps you are working for a short period of time and are unable to leave the office. You can easily bring a breakfast drink. Perhaps you are trying to increase your intake of isoflavones, which are found in soy products, to see if they help with the symptoms of menopause, so you drink soymilk instead of soda.

Make Your Own Dietary Supplements!

- Make your own energy shakes with a partially frozen, vanilla flavored dietary supplement and concentrated orange or grape juice
- Make your own high calcium drink by mixing milk, powdered skim milk powder, vanilla extract, honey or sugar substitute, and your favorite fruit.
- Make peanut butter bars by mixing peanut butter, powdered skim milk or soy powder, and a few drops of honey or water. Roll the balls in your favorite crushed nuts.

Remember, most dietary supplements are high in calories, so eat them sparingly!

Who Is Most Likely to Need or Benefit From Supplements?

- *Iron*—Women with iron deficiency anemia, with heavy menstrual bleeding, infants and small children, persons undergoing rapid growth (like teens)
- *Iron, folate, calcium*—Women that are pregnant or breast feeding
- *Calcium*—Menopausal women
- *Multivitamin with B12 and mineral supplements*—Persons on very low calorie or special diets or vegetarians (see your doctor first)
- *Vitamin D*—Persons with inadequate exposure to sunlight or limited intake of vitamin D fortified milk (see your doctor first)
- *Fluoride*—Some infants and children (must be prescribed, see your doctor first)
- Persons not consuming a healthy diet (see your doctor or Registered Dietitian first to determine your diet and nutrient supplement needs)

Should You Be Taking Vitamin And Mineral Pills or Supplements?

What Should We Ask Ourselves About These Products?
- Do I need this to achieve my goal (be it weight loss, big muscles, energy to function daily, or to have a quick meal)?
- Why am I using this product in place of foods?
- What other alternatives do I have?
- Is this costing me more money than the actual foods?
- What do I stand to gain or lose by not using this product?
- What are the risks associated with using this product?
- Have I come to depend on this as an easy "out" instead of healthier behaviors?
- Do the behaviors promoted by the use of the products reflect my values?

If you are worried about not taking in enough vitamins or minerals, first try to figure out how much you take in through the diet. For example, for calcium, do you have at least three servings of milk and milk products a day? How can you have more milk products or dark, leafy greens? Should you, and how can you, carefully add the use of occasional supplements to your dietary intake of calcium?

Discuss supplements with your doctor. Perhaps there is a medical reason why a supplement is needed. Remember that supplements are precisely that...substances that supplement, **not replace** your usual healthy foods!

Food and Nutrition in This Millennium

There will be many more supplements, especially in pill form, available this millennium. Expect regulations that will standardize these products and provide quality controls. Interestingly enough, as more of them become available, more of them will be marketed as the natural way to eat healthy. But remember, pills are not "natural," and don't expect pills to replace the pleasure and variety that comes from eating foods!

Chapter 7
Combining Traditional, Natural, Convenient, and Functional Foods

There are thousands of foods available in the modern supermarket. Some of these foods, such as an apple or regular (whole) milk, are easy to identify. But it is difficult to identify the ingredients of some foods, such as a meatless hot dog or "fat free" cream cheese.

Commonly Used Terms

There are many terms that are used to describe foods. Some of these terms, such as enriched, organic, or fortified, have legal definitions. Other terms, such as traditional, modern, or convenient, are words that are used by the general population, but they have no legal definition. Some terms, such as refined, are used to refer to a food processing step or function. These terms can mean something different to each person.

Legally Defined and Commonly Accepted Terms

Organically grown or organically produced. According to regulations, the United States Department of Agriculture (USDA) must certify these foods. An organically produced food must be at least 50% organically grown or produced (grown without the use of chemicals, fertilizers, and pesticides). If organically processed, at least 95% of the food must be grown according to federal organic farming standards. These foods cannot contain added sulfites, nitrates, or nitrites.

Functional. "Functional foods," according to the Institute of Medicine, are foods that have been formulated to provide special health benefits. For example, a protein drink for persons on a weight loss diet.

Fortified. Fortified foods have had nutrients added at levels higher than naturally found in the food. In some fortified foods, nutrients have been added that are not found in the original product. For example, most cereals have iron added at levels above those usually found in the product. Folic acid is now also added to certain foods. Fortification must follow Food and Drug Administration (FDA) guidelines. For example, many drinks are fortified with vitamin C.

Enriched. Enrichment is the addition of specific nutrients at a level required to meet a particular standard. The word is generally used to refer to refined breads and cereals, where thiamin, niacin, riboflavin, iron, or folate must be added to replace or supplement the nutrients lost during processing. For example, white flour and bread are enriched.

Dietary supplement. This term is used to mean products made with one or more of the essential nutrients, such as vitamins, minerals, and protein. It also refers to substances extracted from plants, herbs, and botanicals. The word "dietary supplement" must be on the label. A "Supplements Facts" is required on most of these products.

Dietetic foods. This term is used to mean a low calorie or reduced calorie food where an artificial sweetener has been used. This can also be an imitation or modified food that resembles the original food, but is nutritionally inferior. For example, some foods are made with sugar alcohols instead of sugar, and targeted to persons with diabetes.

Medical foods. The terms are often used when referring to beverages or foods such as dietary supplements or tailored foods that are prepared for special health conditions. These words also refer to specially formulated foods, liquid feedings, or formulas that are used in special settings, such as hospitals. Some food scientists prefer to use the word nutraceutical when referring to specially formulated foods (for example, a drink that has been developed for persons that need extra calories and nutrients).

Terms with No Legal Definition

Traditional. There is no formal definition for traditional foods, but the term is generally used to define foods that are historically common to a group. It is assumed that the traditional foods are healthier, more natural, and less processed than convenience foods. However, this assumption may not be correct.

Natural foods. A natural food has been altered as little as possible from its original state. The term commonly means that the food is minimally processed or not at all processed. Some people think that natural foods contain **no** additives, but that is not necessarily so. There is no law that states what can be called natural foods.

Convenience or preprepared. This term is used when referring to foods that have incorporated preparation or serving steps. This may include foods that may be partially or pre-cooked, and only need to be partially prepared or reheated. Food preparation is easier or shorter using these products than if made from scratch.

Refined. This term is used when referring to foods that have had a component, such as the outer covering of a seed, removed. For example, white rice, white flour, and cornstarch are refined foods.

Processed food. This term is used to mean that the food has been modified. It may have been enriched, bleached, milled, or cooked. Almost all foods purchased now have some amount of processing. Non-processed foods are fresh fruits and vegetables, whole grains (like brown rice), and fresh meats, poultry, or fish.

Tailored foods. This term is used for foods that are made for special groups, like a person with diabetes, or special age groups like athletes, infants, or the elderly.

Other terms are also used to describe foods such as modern, designer, synthetic, or formulated. However, these terms are vague and not legally defined. Their definitions and implications, as with many of the already mentioned terms, varies greatly.

CONSUMER TIPS

Confusion with Terms

Do all these definitions or terms seem confusing? Do they seem to overlap? Well, these terms can be confusing, and they do overlap. For example, if you think about it, bread can be called natural, traditional, convenient, refined, or processed. Because there are no legal definitions for some of the terms mentioned, if the sellers want to appeal to your desire for tradition, they may call the bread "traditional." If they want to appeal to your need to ease your busy life, they can call the bread "convenient." If the producers have followed the laws concerning production of organic foods, they can label the bread organic.

Select the Product that is Best for You

As a consumer, what you need to know is *what you want* and *how to get it at the best price.* Do not be fooled by all these food terms. For example, a food may be called natural, but be high in fat or sugar.

Both "natural" and "processed" foods may have positive and negative qualities. Look at the label and compare the ingredients. Then evaluate the calories per serving, fat, and carbohydrates, sugar and other nutrients according to the recommended serving size. That will help you select the product that is best for you.

ISSUES

"Golden Past" Myth

How many times have you heard someone say, "things were better in the past?" In many cases, that may be true. But we also romanticize the past and remember it as better than it was. Do we really want to start making all our foods "from scratch"? Are we willing to make our own bread, tortillas, or cookies? Do we want to peel, slice, and fry our own potatoes *every* time we want French fries? Even if we wanted to do it, would we have the time?

But there are many positive aspects to traditional eating habits. This includes eating together, or eating homemade soups and stews. We want to continue these positive behaviors, but in the context of modern life.

"Newer is Better" Myth

Likewise, you may have heard someone say, "newer is better." There are many positive aspects to modern society, such as vitamin pills, calcium fortified milk, or frozen pizza. But the confusion caused by many new products makes us wish that there would be a slowing down of all that "new" stuff.

It is difficult to generalize and say that "traditional or old" or "modern or new" foods are better. There are healthy foods within each category. For example, traditional foods such as rice, tortillas, bread, oatmeal, and cornmeal are important staples. We should continue to include these foods in our diet. Some modern foods such as calcium fortified milk or calcium fortified orange juice help us increase our intake of a nutrient that is often low in our diets.

CONTEMPORARY LATINO/HISPANIC LIFE

Combining Different Foods

For Latinos/Hispanics, the challenge is to identify healthy traditional and modern foods, and combine them with positive behaviors in our contemporary life.

Some ideas for combining new and traditional foods are:

- Find an easier and healthier way to make a traditional dish such as a *Flan* that uses *egg substitutes,* or eliminate the oil in your stew or soups.

- Add a new ingredient to a traditional dish such as *low-fat turkey sausage* to beans; textured soy protein to a plantain pie or a taco; or a sugar substitute in a fruit shake.

- Learn an easier way to prepare a dish, such as cooking the *chayote* in the *microwave oven,* or using frozen vegetables such as *yuca,* sweet potato, or mixed vegetables in your soups and stews.

- Modernize an old family favorite such as using a vanilla flavored dietary supplement or lactose free milk instead of milk in a *Morir Soñando* or a *batida* (fruit shakes), or substitute lard with sunflower or canola oil.

Ideas for Combining Foods
Main dishes
Put Chinese cabbage in your traditional chicken soup Make your favorite chili with textured soy protein instead of ground beef
Side dishes
Put sun-dried tomatoes in your favorite salad Add bacon flavored soybean crumbles to your salad
Desserts
Put dried cranberries instead of raisins in rice and bread puddings Use the low fat angel food cake for the Tres Leches cake
Snacks
Mix and freeze fresh mashed *mamey* and ice milk for a frozen treat Make tropical fruit shakes with vanilla flavored soymilk

Food and Nutrition in This Millennium

In this millennium, there will be more fortified and functional foods, more supplements, more dietetic, and more tailored foods. Why? Because food producers know that we want foods that have additional nutrients added. They also know that we are looking for easy ways to get more nutrients in our diets. As we worry more about special health conditions or age-related needs, we will want to buy these special foods.

In the future, legal definitions may be developed for some terms, but it is not practical to do so for all food related words. Know what terms have legal definitions. Avoid being misled by words that are used to attract your attention and get your money.

At the same time, as more formulated foods become available, there will be new discoveries of health promoting ingredients in basic foods such as fruits, vegetables, grains, legumes, and nuts. Many of these basic foods are already part of the traditional Latino/Hispanic diet, and will become popular among non-Latinos. Our plantains, *yuca*, sweet potatoes, mangoes, papayas, and other fruits and vegetables are already in vogue among non-Latinos!

Do not let advances in food technology confuse you. It is unlikely that a diet made up primarily of processed foods, even if fortified, will be superior to a diet that is primarily composed of basic foods. Benefit from the new technologies by **focusing on basic foods and using the formulated products to enhance your basic diet.**

Chapter 8

Contemporary Latinos/Hispanics: Smart Consumers and Cooks

Food Expenses

Latinos/Hispanics in the United States have a purchasing power of over $350 billion dollars per year. But do we spend that money wisely? It is a good idea to know how much of our income is spent on food. However, how much we spend on food is not the only indicator of whether or not we are spending our money wisely. Sometimes the percent we spend on food is high because the *income is low*, but sometimes the percent we spend on food is high because food expenses are *not well planned*.

One easy way to determine what percent of our money is spent on food is to divide how much we spend on food (including meals eaten out) by our net income. For example:

- Net Income: $500.00

- Estimated total spent on food: $100.00 ($75.00 groceries + $25 eating out)

- Percent spent on food = 100/500 X 100 = 20%

Notice that this family is spending 20% of the net income on food. The U.S. average is 10%-15%. There can be various reasons why this family's is spending 20%. For example, perhaps the net income is low, or the family is not spending the food money wisely.

In either case, the important question that the family may want to discuss is "Are we making the best use of our food money?" There are various ways to achieve this goal, but regardless of the methods used, it is very important that all family members eat well.

Planning and Shopping Guidelines

Here are ten quick and easy steps for planning and shopping that can help you save money on your food bill.

1. Identify what you have at home.

2. Plan a menu around the foods that you have at home (include snacks and foods for work or school). Planning a menu does not have to be complicated. Make a mental picture of what family members will be eating for meals, snacks, and at school or work.

3. Identify the things you need.

4. Write a shopping list. Incorporate healthy foods that are on sale, seasonal foods, and store or generic brands.

5. Go shopping **on a full stomach,** not when you are hungry. Avoid impulsive selections.

6. Only use coupons for items that you commonly use.

7. Stick to your shopping list, unless you find a less costly substitute.

8. Buy meat according to the number of servings per pound, not by cost per pound.

9. Buy fruits and vegetables in season.

10. Buy canned and frozen fruits and vegetables when on sale.

Do a quick check of the nutritional value of your menu and purchases by asking yourself the following questions:

Question	Yes/No/Add
1. Does this menu include grains, breads, or other starchy food at **each** meal?	
2. Does this menu include fruits and/or juice **two or three** times a day?	
3. Does this menu include vegetables (alone or in foods) or salads **two or three** times a day?	
4. Does this menu include dairy products such as skim milk, cheeses, or yogurt, **two or three** times a day?	
5. Does this menu include egg, meat, fish, beans, or nuts, **twice** a day?	
6. Do I have "other" foods (such as chips, soda, oil, etc.)? How can I substitute them with healthier foods?	
7. Do I have supplements (such as weight loss shakes, etc.)? Are they worth the cost, or can I achieve my goal by just eating less or by choosing wisely among the basic items?	

Understanding Food Labels

Food labels provide a lot of information that can help us decide if we want to buy a product. When looking at food labels, carefully read the *name* of the product, the *size*, the *form*, the *ingredients* (if listed) and the *nutrition information*. Let's look at the nutrition information on a label and identify the ways that we can use this information.

Basic Information	
1. Name of product (and form or description, if necessary).	
2. Weight, measure, or count.	
3. Name and address of the manufacturer, packer, or distributor.	
4. Ingredients in descending order by weight (unless they have a standard of identity).	

Nutrition Information

Nutrition information is available on the Nutrition Facts section of almost all products. This panel has two parts. The top part has information specific to the food package. The bottom part has reference information that is based on Daily Values for a 2,000 calorie diet. The Daily Values are the reference values developed by the United States Food and Drug Administration for use on food labels.

The Top Portion of the Food Label

1.	Standard serving size in common household and metric measure.
2.	Number of servings or portions per package.
3.	Total calories (energy) per serving.
4.	Fat grams per serving (and a breakdown of the grams of saturated fat and milligrams of cholesterol).
5.	Sodium, in milligrams, per serving.
6.	Carbohydrates, in grams, per serving.
7.	Fiber and sugar, in grams, per serving.
8.	Protein, in grams, per serving.
9.	Amount of Vitamins A and C, as a percentage of the Daily Values for 2,000 calories per day.
10.	Minerals, calcium and iron, as a percentage of the Daily Values for 2,000 calories per day.

The Bottom Portion of the Food Label

The bottom portion of the label provides information on the Daily Values based on a 2,000 and 2,500 calorie diet.

Five Terms You Want to Know

1. "Free" = nutritionally trivial, without, or zero amount.

2. "High" = 20% or more of the Daily Value, rich in, or an excellent source of a given nutrient.

3. "Light" = one third fewer calories than the comparison food or, for fats, 50% or less fat than the comparison food.

4. "Sodium free" = less than 5 mg. sodium per serving.

5. "Cholesterol free" = less than 2 mg. cholesterol, and 2 grams or less of saturated fat per serving.

Some of the Ways We Can Use the Information on a Label

Use	Example
To compare two of the same, or similar, products.	Canned beans: 1. Two different brands of canned black beans. 2. A can of black beans packed in water and a can of black bean soup. **Tip:** Compare the **prices** and how you will **use** the product.
To compare the calories per serving sizes.	Two frozen pizzas, both 12 ounces: 1. 240 calories, 2 ounces each serving size, 6 servings per package. 2. 180 calories per serving size, 1.5 ounces, 8 servings per package. **Tip:** Compare the individual **serving sizes**. Is the smaller size too small, and are you likely to eat two slices? That's 360 calories!
To compare the nutrient values.	Two different frozen vegetables, such as green beans and carrots: 1. One serving of the green beans has 10% of the daily value for Vitamin A. 2. One serving of the carrots has 110% of the daily value for Vitamin A. **Tip:** For nutrient variety, purchase different fruits and vegetables with **at least** 20%-25% of a specific nutrient such as carrots, which are high in Vitamin A, and canned pineapple, which is high in Vitamin C.
To determine the ratio of nutrient to calories.	Two different beverages, such as whole milk and soda: 1. Whole milk has 180 calories and 33% of the daily value for calcium (180:33). 2. Cola has 180 calories and 0% of the daily value for calcium (180:0). This is an "empty-calorie" beverage. **Tip:** Select beverages that provide **nutritional value for their calories**. Avoid the "empty-calorie" beverages.

Preparation, Use, and Storage

If you purchase healthy foods but prepare them improperly or waste them, you will have lost nutrients, time, and money. Here are a few preparation, use and storage tips:

Grains, Breads, Starches

1. Make your own pre-prepared mixes such as chicken broth cubes, rice, peas or lentils; add your favorite seasonings, and freeze the mixture in plastic freezer bags.
2. Cook large amounts of rice and freeze portions of it in plastic freezer bags.
3. Roll large tortillas with lean cold cuts, wrap tightly in plastic wrap and freeze. Heat them in the microwave oven for a quick snack or lunch.
4. Eliminate or decrease the oil usually added to rice or pasta.
5. To avoid spoilage and retain moistness, freeze breads that you do not plan to use within 2 or 3 days.

Fruits

1. Freeze individual juice packs and use them as an ice pack in a bag with a sandwich.
2. Wash fruit and keep it near the door. That way you can grab one on the way to work or school.
3. Mix juices with diet ginger ale or flavored, calorie free waters.
4. Mix different flavor juices for a nutritious drink (like pineapple juice and apricot nectar for a high vitamin C and vitamin A juice).
5. Use juices in recipes (like apple juice in *Flan*, or pineapple juice in a cake mix).

Vegetables

1. Purchase premixed salad packs and tomatoes for a quick salad.
2. Sprinkle vegetables such as broccoli or *chayote*, with grated cheese, and cook them in the microwave oven.

3. Cook potatoes in the microwave oven for a quick lunch or to add to other dishes. This way you do not have to fry the potatoes and get all those extra calories.

4. When on sale, buy cans or frozen packages of vegetables for serving, or as an addition to rice, pasta, soups, or stews.

5. Add diced or small pieces of your leftover vegetables to cooked rice or stews.

6. Keep jars of spaghetti or marinara sauce for a quick sauce or seasoning base.

Dairy Products

1. Keep unflavored, plain yogurt and use it instead of, or mixed with, sour cream (especially for *quesadillas* or *tacos*).

2. Premix powdered dry skim milk and sugar or sugar substitute, and keep at home or work for your coffee.

3. If you do not tolerate milk well, use a "lactose-free" or "low-lactose" milk as a beverage and in cooking.

4. Cut your favorite cheese into cubes and wrap tightly. Place the cheese cubes in small bags with wrapped crackers, and have them handy for lunch or a snack.

5. Buy powdered or canned evaporated milk for use in prepared dishes or desserts.

Meat and Meat Substitutes

1. Preseason meats with garlic, pepper, dried herbs (not salt) and freeze them in plastic freezer bags.

2. Cook large amounts of meats and freeze them in individual servings in plastic freezer bags.

3. Precook meat in the microwave prior to baking, broiling, grilling or barbecuing.

4. Boil chicken prior to freezing. You can quickly thaw it in the microwave oven, dice it, and put it in your favorite dishes.

5. Freeze the broth from the boiled chicken in an ice cube tray. Use the cubes to sauté meats or vegetables. Use the broth instead of oil. This will save money and reduce the caloric intake as well.

6. Cut down on the cost of the meat by preparing mixed dishes with rice and pasta, and small amounts of meat.

7. Pick up pre-prepared broiled or baked chicken and serve it with the previously cooked rice that you had frozen, and the pre-mixed salad.

8. Use meat substitutes such as cheese, beans, eggs, or soy with meals.

Other Foods

1. Make your own low salt/low sodium seasoning mix by combining garlic power, onion powder, pepper, paprika, cumin, turmeric, or curry powder and other seasonings. Did you know that the commercial ones are as much as 90% salt?

2. Make your own flavoring bases such as *salsa or recaito*, freeze them in an ice cube tray, and store the frozen cubes in plastic freezer bags.

3. Make sandwiches with mustard and lean cold meats. Freeze them in tightly sealed sandwich bags. Take the sandwich to work with your frozen juice pack.

4. Mix nonfat cream cheese, nuts, and honey or diced fruit (like pineapple) or vegetables (like peppers, carrots or celery), for a quick low calorie spread.

5. Make snack packs with your favorite dry cereal, nuts, and dried fruits.

6. Make low calorie frozen desserts by mixing ice milk and diced or pureed fruit (such as chopped pineapple) and freezing it for future use.

CONSUMER TIPS

What Type Of A Food Shopper Are You?

There are different types of shopping styles. You may have one shopping style or change your style depending on the amount of time you have available.

- Some persons walk around the store's periphery. They tend to run around the periphery of the store, just picking up the basics.

- Some persons dip into or "spot" aisles. They are the persons that block your entry to the aisle. They are standing at the entrance trying to determine if there is something that they need.

- Some persons "weave" or walk up and down each aisle.

As a weaver, you will usually spend more time and more money. Some supermarkets try to get you to weave or spend a lot of time at the store with the soft paced music and attractive displays. They may place basic foods such as bread in hard to find areas. Try to become a peripheral or spot shopper. The peripheral shopper tends to buy the basic items because these foods are usually found in those areas of supermarkets.

The "Shopping Game"
Think of food shopping as a game. *How fast* can you come in and out of the store with *only* the necessary items?

1. Figure out where the basic foods (milk, eggs, fruits, vegetables, rice, bread, etc.) are located.
2. Plan out the easiest and fastest way to walk through the store to get to these foods.
3. Identify and avoid unnecessary areas and items that are a waste of money.
4. Look up and down the shelves. The lower priced and less popular brands are often placed above or below eye level.

Remember: You generally pay less for the less processed foods and the larger sizes. But this is not always the case. It is not a *sale* if you do not use the food or it spoils. You just lost money.

ISSUES

Additives: Are They Good or Bad?

Most persons think that additives are either "good" or "bad." But it is more useful to know some basic information about additives. First, there are two major classifications of additives: the intentional and the non-intentional. Second, each classification has several subcategories. Third, most additives have very useful functions. Fourth, the more processed a food is, the more additives it will have.

Intentional Additives

Intentional additives are classified according to, and added to, foods for a specific purpose. For example:

- Preservatives—help foods last longer
- Added Nutrients—serve as nutrients for the body (such as Vitamin C when added to foods)
- Emulsifiers—keep foods, such as oil and vinegar, from separating
- Antioxidants—keep food from becoming rancid or spoiled
- Flavor enhancers—give additional flavor to the food
- Coloring agents—give or enhance the color of a food
- Antimicrobials—keep germs from growing on foods
- Bleaching agents—help whiten or give even color to foods
- Thickeners—help make a food thicker

Some of these additives are familiar to us, such as cornstarch, which is used to thicken food. Some of us may already do this at home. Some additives are naturally found in food. For example lecithin, which occurs naturally in egg yolk, is used in the food industry to keep foods from separating, such as oil and vinegar. Other additives, such as sodium carbonate, are not generally used at home.

Non-Intentional Additives

Non-intentional additives appear in food as a result of growing, harvesting, handling, preparing, or packaging. This can range from a piece of paper to a pesticide. Some non-intentional additives may be harmful. Obviously, we prefer not to have these types of additives in foods. Nevertheless, the goal is to avoid non-intentional additives. This is done by setting standards of quality and enforcing them. As a consumer, you want to buy items from companies that have high standards in the handling and preparation of foods.

There is concern that we are consuming too many additives. Many of us worry that their frequent and/or long-term use might be harmful. As well, some persons may have sensitivities to certain additives. A personal goal might be to try to consume as few additives as possible. One way that we can do this is to avoid eating too many processed foods.

Non Nutrients in Food: Caffeine

We eat many non-nutrients, such as caffeine, sugar substitutes, and phytochemicals. Some of these non-nutrients, like the phytochemicals, may be desirable. Others are beneficial because they give foods unique characteristics like texture, color, or flavor. But others may be harmful. The most common non-nutrient, which is also considered a drug, is caffeine.

Caffeine is found in coffee, tea, chocolate, sodas, and some over-the-counter medications. It stimulates the central nervous system, so it helps alertness. But it can raise blood pressure and stimulate urination. Excessive caffeine intake can cause headaches and increase the heartbeat. Too much caffeine may make it difficult to concentrate, and cause sweating, or tenseness. If you or your children drink coffee, colas, and eat chocolate every day, you are probably taking in more caffeine than is desirable.

We should try to limit our adult intake of caffeine to a range of 200 to 300 mg. a day. Avoid giving it to children. Adults can have one cup of coffee and then drink decaffeinated coffee, juices, and water throughout the day. Eat a carob bar instead of a chocolate bar once in a while. Carob is a popular chocolate substitute.

Caffeine Content of Some Common Foods			
Food	Caffeine Level (mg)	Range (mg)	Comments
Coffee, drip, "American style" 5 ounces	115	40—180	Many places serve more than 5 ounces.
Coffee, espresso, 2 ounces	100	40—170	Many persons drink more than 2 ounces.
Tea, brewed, 5 ounces	40	20—110	Imported brands tend to have more caffeine than US brands. Iced tea is about a 12 ounce serving.
Sodas, 12 ounces	35	35—60	Some newer drinks have extra caffeine added.
Milk chocolate bar, 1 ounce	5	5—35	Darker chocolate is higher in caffeine.

Food Safety

Most persons, when asked about food safety, think about additives or pesticides. But, the most common food related danger has to do with germs in food. Germs are living organisms, just like us. So, depending on the germ, a temperature between 40 to 140 degrees Fahrenheit is a "danger zone." That is the temperature range at which germs will grow most rapidly. Germs can double in numbers in just **20 minutes!**

The microorganisms are small but have long names. Salmonella, Escheria Coli (E. coli), Staphylococcus Aureus (Staph), Campylobacter, Clostridium Perfringens, Clostridium Botulinum, Listeria Monocytogenes,

Shigella, and Vibrio Vulnificus cause most of the food infections or food poisonings. These germs are transmitted through raw, undercooked, or uncooked foods. Or they may grow on a food that was well cooked but left out to cool.

Food Safety Tips
- **Keep the Kitchen Clean:** Wash hands frequently, disinfect work surfaces, appliances, sponges and cloths. Add two teaspoons of bleach to one quart of water to make a disinfecting solution.
- **Keep Items Separate:** Many of us use the same cutting board for meats and other foods, or the same spoon to stir then taste food, or serve food with our eating utensil. Use different equipment or wash it thoroughly with hot soapy water between uses. Don't cross contaminate foods (that is, using the same knife for cutting raw meat, then using it for cutting vegetables which will be used in a salad.)
- **Have Errands to Run?** Buy food last, or bring a cooler with ice and put the meats and other cold foods in the cooler.
- **Thaw and Cool Foods Correctly.** Do not leave food on the counter to thaw or to cool or to wait for others to eat. If you leave food out at room temperature, germs will grow very quickly!
- **Cook Foods Thoroughly.** This will help avoid food poisoning or illness by destroying germs through cooking.

The general rule is to *keep cold foods cold* (below 40 degrees F) and *hot foods hot* (above 140 F). Remember if it feels "nice and warm" to you, it is a great growing temperature for germs.

If you are not sure a food is safe to eat, ___do not taste it.___ (Think about that. Isn't it kind of silly? Yet, that is the first thing many of us do.) ___Throw it out!___ Children, the elderly, or already ill persons, are especially at greater risk for illness. See a doctor if there is fever, vomiting, or bloody stools. Although rare, C. botulinum and Listeria can be fatal.

CONTEMPORARY LATINO/HISPANIC LIFE

Frequent eating out and consumption of convenience foods mark contemporary Latino/Hispanic life. These foods may be handled multiple times by many different people, or they may be left standing for long periods of time. As a result, the likelihood of food illness is increased. In addition to practicing high food safety standards at home, demand them at commercial establishments.

Food and Nutrition in This Millennium

This millennium will bring us more shopping options than ever before. We will buy foods in large supermarkets, small, gourmet, and specialty stores, and through the Internet!

There will also be more forms of a food available. We will be able to buy foods fresh, canned, dehydrated, irradiated, powdered, partially cooked, instant, and in many other forms. This will make shopping a very confusing activity. We will need to know all these market forms and evaluate their prices.

This millennium we will need more shopping and evaluation skills than ever before. If we can use these skills effectively, we will be able to select wisely and enjoy foods from thousands of choices.

Chapter 9
The Life Cycle: Eating Well Throughout Your Life

Introduction

Although *eating* is one of our basic and lifelong activities, we will have different *nutritional* needs at different stages in our life. Understanding what these needs are, and eating to meet them, will help us improve the quality of our life.

Do you know that your health *now* was influenced by your grandparents' health? Yes, how well your grandmother took care of herself in some part impacted you. Likewise, the grandchild or great grandchild that you have not seen or perhaps even dreamt about will be influenced by how you are eating *now*.

Infants and Toddlers—Up to Two Years

Can you imagine yourself as an adult tripling in weight and doubling in height within one year? Yet, that is roughly the growth that an infant will experience during the first year! Babies grow so rapidly in this stage of their lives that they need more vitamin A, C, and D, iron, zinc, calcium, and other nutrients now than at any other time in their lives. That is why babies are eating and growing machines!

Breast-feeding Is Best

Interestingly, in the United States, Latino/Hispanic mothers from South America or those that have recently come to the U.S. are more likely to breast-feed than those that came from the Caribbean Islands or have been in the U.S. for a while. But we do not know why this is so.

Perhaps it is because some persons believe that formula feeding is the modern, more convenient, or economical thing to do. But, it's important for us to remember that in this case, *what's old is what's new*. Why? Because we know that, except in very rare circumstances, mother's milk is the *best* milk for an infant child. It provides the right nutrients and in amounts that the child needs. A healthy mother's milk **changes over time** to adjust to the infant's nutritional needs.

Mother's milk contains immunoglobulins. These substances help the infant fight diseases. Breast-fed children have fewer colds, infections, and allergies than formula-fed children. It appears that breast-fed babies are less likely to develop some diseases, such as diabetes and cancer in later life. If you are breast-feeding, ask your doctor if you need to give your baby vitamin and mineral supplements (iron, fluoride, and vitamin D).

For Moms, breast-feeding is a time for bonding and relaxing (and you will definitely feel you need to relax!). Breast-feeding is not difficult. It does not require mixing formulas, cleaning and sanitizing bottles and nipples, refrigeration, or as much shopping as formula feeding. It helps Mom regain her flat abdomen by stimulating uterine contractions. If you eat well and drink plenty of fluids, breast-feeding is also more economical than formula feeding.

But When Should You Use Infant Formula?

It is usually better to give the baby mother's milk. For the first twelve months of life, breast milk or formula provide your baby with most of his or her nutrient needs. If you cannot breastfeed for a long period of time, breast-feed for at least the first few days after the baby's birth, or as long as possible. During the first few days, your milk will provide the baby with colostrum, which has the substances that help protect against infections.

If you must return to work, or want others to help you with feeding the baby, express and transfer your breast milk into a bottle. That way the infant can still drink your milk. You can get more information and help for this from the local La Leche League or call a lactation consultant. If you need to totally wean the infant, change the child from breast milk to infant formula, **not** cow's milk. If you are ill, especially with a contagious illness or are not available during feeding times, give the infant *formula* **not** cow's milk. Whole milk can be given **after** the baby is over one year of age.

What is in That Diaper?
Did you know that a breastfed baby has a looser stool than a formula fed baby? This is okay. It occurs because the breast milk is easier to digest than formula!

How About Other Foods?

Introduce solid foods when the baby is about 4-6 months old. First give the baby plain, single ingredient foods. For example, start with rice cereal, then barley, and then corn. Introduce wheat cereal last. When introducing a new food, wait about three days and watch for diarrhea or a skin rash, which might be a sign of a food allergy or food sensitivity.

First, give the baby the fortified cereals. About 5 months, begin to add pureed vegetables such as peas, and then carrots. Then add fruits, such as applesauce and peaches. A few months later, add pureed or finely chopped meats and poultry, as well as cooked dried beans and peas, which have been mashed. As the infant nears one year of age, offer a variety of whole grain breads, crackers, yogurt, and cheese. Wait until the baby is one year of age before giving him or her egg whites, as they can cause an allergy to eggs in some infants.

To help the infant accept new foods, offer the same food for several days and at different times. Learning to eat a variety of foods helps set the stage for life-long healthful eating habits and acceptance of a variety of foods. Remember that after one year of age, eating only one food is not healthy.

Tips for Introducing New Foods	
At about 4-6 months (baby can sit with help and hold his/her head without support):	• Start with single grain iron-fortified cereals mixed with mother's milk or formula. • Suggested order: rice cereal, oat, or barley. Introduce wheat cereal last.
At about 6-7 months (baby sits without help and can put food in mouth):	• Follow with single strained vegetables (squash, peas, mashed potatoes, etc.). • Add strained fruits and strained, unsweetened juices. • Introduce strained vegetables before fruits, so that the child doesn't get used to the sweet taste and reject the vegetables.
At about 7-9 months (baby can bite food and pick up small pieces):	• Introduce soft breads, teething biscuits, crackers. • Give textured vegetables and fruits. • Give unsalted strained meats and egg yolk.
At about 10-12 months (baby can use a spoon and baby cup):	• Gradually start on finely chopped meats, fish, soft cheeses. • Serve dry unsweetened cereals, rice, pasta, mashed legumes. • Give yogurts, soft cheeses. • Give whole eggs when the baby is one year old.

Important Reminders About Your Tiny Eating Machine!
- Occasionally give water; 1 to 2 ounces, especially in hot climates.
- Don't introduce solids too early (before four months). Their digestive system is not ready, and the baby may have an allergic reaction to the food.
- Avoid concentrated sweets; they may cause diarrhea and obesity.
- Avoid honey as it may cause botulism, a potentially fatal disease.
- Avoid corn syrup as a sweetener; a large concentration may cause diarrhea.
- Feed solids from a spoon—not from a baby bottle-type feeder.
- About **one** tablespoon of each food is an adequate serving size for a young baby.
- Serve from a dish, not the jar, to avoid contamination.
- Remember, if you add salt to *your taste*, it's too salty for the baby.
- Do not chew the baby's food before giving it to him or her!!

Growing Up

After the first year of life, the rate of growth slows down. The interest in food decreases and the interest in the other things (such as play) increases. **Don't force the child to eat.** It is important to remember that the child's appetite will decrease as a result of the decreased rate of growth.

The toddler is becoming more independent. This "little person" now enjoys self-feeding and has individual food likes and dislikes, and food jags are common. A food jag is an eating pattern in which the child seems to want the same food all the time! Toddlers may choose these favorite foods for a period of time, and then ignore them. Since food jags are usually short term, toddlers' nutrient intakes are balanced over time. Do not worry about the jag; merely serve a variety of foods *along* with the favorite item.

Your child will want to eat small amounts of food throughout the day. Space meals and snacks, but provide structured, regular eating times. Don't worry if the child does not want to eat all the food. Serve small amounts. Generally a child will stop eating once he or she is full (unlike some adults!).

Foods After the First Year of Age

After one year of age, give the child about four glasses of whole milk (1/2 cup at a time) each day, to be certain that the child gets enough calcium. We should not give them low fat milks prior to two years of age, because they need the extra fat calories for growth. After age two, gradually switch from whole milk to low fat or skim milk.

If sodas, fruit drinks, or juices are offered in place of milk, the child will likely not get enough calcium and some other minerals needed for growth.

Portion Sizes

A toddler's portion is about 1/4 to 1/3 the size of an adult portion (less if you are a family of big eaters!). A general guide for a serving size, or portion for a child, is one tablespoon of each food for every year of age. Encourage children to *sit and eat until they are full*, to tell you they are full, and ask for permission to leave the table. This avoids over feeding. Avoid using food (especially sweets) as a reward.

Sample Menu for a 2-3 Year-Old Toddler	
1/4 cup	Peas.
1/4 cup	Rice.
1/4 - 1/3 cup	Diced chicken.
1/2 glass	Milk.

Remember, generally a toddler only *needs* about 1-2 ounces of meat. That is about 1/4 or 1/3 of a commercial burger. So if you order a burger for your toddler, be HAPPY if he or she eats 1/3 of the burger. Don't force the child to eat the rest! You may share the hamburger instead of ordering two if you want to eat less as well.

> Toddlers learn most through modeling. You are their idol, so watch what and how much you eat, and how you behave at the table!

Make eating fun. (Do you remember being punished because you would not eat your meat? Didn't you promise yourself you would not do that to *your* children?) What can you do to make eating fun for them and easier for you? Here are a few tips:

1. Ask the child to help you plan the meal. She/he may come up with new, fun ideas!

2. Cut or shape food in funny ways (serve rice in a heart shape, trim the tortillas edges to simulate sunshine). Have the child help you, if possible.

3. Let the child make up a name for a dish. Put a nametag on the table next to the dish.

4. Have "special meal days" for family members. Others can help make the special meal, including the toddler. For example, on "Samuel's Saturday," have the toddler help make a special food for Samuel.

5. Let the child help you clean. This is a great time to get the child started on that habit!

Children

Your school-age child has already developed food habits that were learned at home. The person that spent large amounts with the toddler influenced that child the most. It is the same at school. Your school-aged child will now be interested in learning from classmates and other authority figures such as teachers, principals, and their friend's parents. Don't be upset about that. However, be careful to know and regulate from whom your child is learning these new behaviors. You may want to find out:

1. If a variety of foods are served at school, and if menus are based on nutritional guidelines.
2. If there are easily accessible facilities for food service employees and children to wash their hands.
3. If the school's food preparation areas are clean.
4. If other instruction and preparation areas (such as a lab) are kept clean and separate from the food preparation areas.
5. How these other people feel about food and food behaviors.

The years from 5-12 are a good age to teach children about the relationship between health and food choices. They are learning different subjects, and this will help them link or see relationships between topics. This will help them learn and value the consequences of behavior and help them prepare for the future. Use a positive approach and make learning fun!

Quick Breakfasts

Mornings are a hectic time in just about every household. It is difficult to prepare full breakfast meals. Sometimes we even skip meals. But if we got up and ran to school without breakfast, by midmorning we would be too tired and weak to be very productive. This can have a negative impact on a child's learning. A hungry or tired child has trouble listening, concentrating, and behaving. Irritability may be a sign of hunger.

What are some easy breakfast foods? There are many items that we can make quickly or prepare in advance and store in the freezer or refrigerator.

> **Easy Breakfast Foods for Busy Kids and Their Parents**
>
> Serve any of the following with a glass of milk or juice:
> - A piece of Italian bread with some *queso blanco* and guava jelly.
> - Cheese and/or ham wrapped in a tortilla.
> - Dry cereal in small plastic bags.
> - Cold left over chicken breast.
> - Yogurt with fruit.
> - A pre-cooked, cold, hard cooked egg.
> - A pre-prepared ham sandwich.
> - Mashed beans wrapped in a tortilla.
> - A bagel with a slice of cheddar cheese.
> - A piece of Spanish style bread pudding.

Healthy School Lunches

One of the biggest concerns I have is packed lunches. Some caregivers do not have their children eat lunch at school because they do not consider school meals nutritious. However, it is not unusual for a child to bring to school a meal that includes a *bologna sandwich, potato chips, cookies or candy, and a soda or fruit drink.* This is a high fat, high sodium, high added sugar meal.

Food safety in home prepared lunches is also a concern. Imagine a bologna sandwich, prepared at 7 in the morning, in an unrefrigerated school bag until 12 noon. That stomachache and mild diarrhea later in the day may be the result of food poisoning or food infection, not a cold!

Healthy, Great Tasting, Economical, and Safe Choices!
- Lean cuts of meat—Chicken, turkey, and ham sandwiches. Freeze sandwiches; pack frozen.
- Economical items—peanut butter, cheese sandwiches, leftover cuts of meat. Put leftover rice and beans, leftover meat or chicken, or homemade soups in a hot thermos.
- Beverages—Freeze commercial brick packs of 100% mixed juices and pack them with your sandwich in your lunch bag to keep the sandwich or other foods cold.
- Snack items—Pack fruits such as applesauce, grapes, bananas, apples, oranges, peaches, in plastic containers. Pack cookies that are low fat or fruit filled (not fruit-*flavored*), peanuts, sunflower seeds, unsalted pretzels, or popcorn.

Obesity

How many times have you heard someone say "What a pretty, fat, baby!" Obesity is a growing problem among our children. As many as 1/5th of children are overweight. While there are many causes for obesity, in general, it is combination of eating too much, and not being very active.

In some cases, a child may become mildly deficient in specific nutrients due to poor eating habits, such as eating too much of the wrong foods (like sodas, chips, and sweets). Or, the child may drink too much milk throughout the day. Remember, milk is very good because it is high in calcium, but it is also low in iron. If a child drinks too much milk, and he or she does not eat enough of the other foods, such as meat, green vegetables, or beans, the child may develop iron deficiency anemia, even though he or she may be fat.

What If Your Child Is Getting Too Fat?

1. Encourage physical activity...**not dieting!** Help the child "grow" into his or her weight.

2. Purchase healthy low calorie snacks for the home and school.

3. Encourage "trading" unhealthy choices for healthier ones, such as a small orange juice and a plain burger instead of a soda and a "fancy" burger.

4. Serve smaller portions, and don't encourage seconds.

5. Teach the child to compare calories and fat on food labels and to prepare "lower calorie" alternatives. This will greatly help the child when he or she is an adult.

Teenagers

Accept it. Once your child becomes a teenager, it is very difficult to control his or her food habits. That's why what he or she learned from you in the earlier years, when you were the idol, is so very important. Now their idols will be movie stars, other teenagers, or even a favorite teacher.

Probably the most important thing you can do to promote healthy eating is to keep open the lines of communication. In all likelihood, many of your teenagers' daily activities will not include you. So you won't know what they eat most of the time, unless you take the time to have pleasant conversation with them.

Nutritional Needs of Teenagers

Teenagers are going through a growth spurt. This is an important period of growth because their bodies are preparing them for their reproductive and later years. Girls' growth generally peaks at about 12 years. Boys' growth generally peaks at about 14 years. But it is not unusual for growth to peak earlier or later (much to the concern of the teenager that is feeling "different").

The need for most nutrients increases during adolescence. Females will have an increased need for iron due to menstruation. More calcium is needed for males and females because bone growth (that is, depositing calcium in bones) will continue into their 20s. There is usually an increase in activities (especially in males), which demands more energy (calories).

There will be many physical changes in the teenager, and the physical growth will usually not correspond to the emotional or social growth. Think of the "big" teenage baby boy in your family. Or maybe there is a physically undeveloped girl that already acts like a young lady! These are difficult years, and sometimes food is the last thing the teenager is worried about, even though it may concern you!

Often, if the teenager *is* concerned about food, it's related to wanting to lose or gain weight. Food is just a means to achieving a desired body or look. Help your child have realistic ideas and goals about their desired body look. Then, don't argue. Work with him or her to achieve that goal in a healthy way.

To Gain Weight...or to Build the Body?

Find out if the goal is to lose weight or to build the body. If the goal is to build the body, help the teenager develop a muscle building regimen. Help the teenager identify some muscle, chest, waist, or leg exercises, and a safe schedule for increasing the exercises.

Work with the teenager to identify healthy beverages and foods for the exercise routines. For example, prepare a large pitcher of diluted juice and water. The teenager can drink this before, during, and after the activity. Have crackers, pretzels, and fruits available for before and after the activity.

Discuss the uses, potential harmful effects, and excessive cost of body building supplements. For example, amino acid supplements are unnecessary if you are eating enough protein. Also, taking in too many amino acids is stressful on the kidneys, which must act to clear the body of the amino acid wastes. There are many foods that we already eat, and can enjoy, that have very good amino acid combinations (such as eggs, beans and tortillas, rice and beans, chicken, fish, milk, beef, pork, cheese, powdered skim milk, and tuna).

Remind the teenager that steroids cause side effects such as acne, aggressive behavior, and damage to the testes, all the things that will make them unattractive. Steroids are also illegal.

To Lose Weight

It has been estimated that as many as 80% of 5th grade girls have been on a diet. Girls are dieting before they even become teenagers. As more teenage girls are lured by the images on television and other media, they come to believe that to be beautiful they must be very tall and thin. But in reality, very few women are naturally very tall and thin. So, this unrealistic expectation about beauty can become very frustrating, especially for Latino women, many of whom are petite and fuller bodied.

Try to help your teenage daughter be comfortable about her natural body without encouraging her to be obese or obsessive about losing weight. Point out role models of smaller, petite teen idols. Help her set realistic weight goals and ways to improve her self-esteem and appearance that do not involve weight. Then help her find ways to achieve the goals. This may include physical activities such as soccer, dancing, a martial art, tennis, basketball, or softball. These activities are a healthy way to lose weight and become physically fit. This is a positive health behavior that she can carry into later life. In this millennium, adults, including the elderly, will lead healthy, active lives, and you will have helped her prepare for such.

Tips for Teens	
In A Hurry? Have:	**Out With Friends? Pick:**
• Chocolate milk • Bagel with a slice of cheese	• (Any) fruit juice • Pizza with onions, mushrooms, or other veggies
• Fruit flavored yogurt • Banana or other fruit	• Char grilled chicken • Tossed salad
• Ham and cheese sandwich • A 100% mixed fruit juice	• Baked apple pie • Low fat milk
• Cold piece of chicken (not fried) • Chocolate milk	• Turkey sandwich • Decaffeinated skim milk latte

Adults

Did you know that we may continue to deposit calcium in our bones until we are about 30? The body is trying to make our bones dense and prepare us for our calcium needs in later life. Although adults have reached physiological maturity, the body still needs nutrients to maintain body functions and replace tissues.

As in our teenage years, we tend to be active in our young adult years. This means we can often "afford" to eat many calories, because we are using them up. However, over time we tend to become less active. We may take on more sedentary jobs. We participate in fewer sports, go dancing less frequently, and start watching more television. In addition, as we grow older, we start to earn more money, buy more foods, eat out more, and get fatter!

The adult years are often ignored in terms of diet and health. But these are very important years for practicing behaviors that will minimize the risk for hypertension, diabetes, heart disease, cancer, and other diseases in later life.

What should you be watching out for? Care for yourself by:

1. Avoiding weight gain. Think about it. If you are within an acceptable weight range at age 20 and gain just two pounds a year, you will be about 40 pounds overweight by the time you are 40, and 80 pounds overweight at age 60, before you even retire!

2. Avoiding high fat and high sodium foods. High fat intake is a risk factor for heart disease and cancer. High sodium intake is a risk factor for hypertension for sodium-sensitive persons.

3. Eating lots of fruits, vegetables, and beans. We keep identifying phytochemicals in these foods that seem to help protect us against many diseases.

4. Consuming high calcium foods, especially if you have a family history of osteoporosis.

5. Consuming plenty of foods rich in iron, especially if you are a female or a vegetarian. Women often have insufficient iron intakes. Eat beans, dark greens, and cook in iron pots.

6. Consuming alcohol in moderation. Cirrhosis of the liver is often caused by excessive alcohol intake. It is a debilitating disease that can be prevented through moderate consumption.

Women's Unique Problems

Is your blood pressure high? Are you at risk for breast cancer or heart disease? High blood pressure, heart disease, and cancer, are women's issues. They are not just men's issues. Remember, you cannot care for your family if you are ill. Take time to care for your health, so you can be in an emotional and physical state to take care of others. There are a few issues that an adult female faces that are unique to her role as mother and wife. These issues relate to her social role or her special physiological needs.

From a social perspective, some Hispanic women may be so concerned with their family's health that they neglect their own. For example, some women with iron deficiency anemia do not prepare a high iron food that is important for and liked by them (such as chicken livers) because the family members do not like it! Women with iron deficiency anemia need to consult their doctor or Registered Dietitian for information about iron supplements and high iron foods.

If you are pregnant, at risk for osteoporosis, or have iron deficiency anemia, you have special dietary needs that must be addressed. Pregnant women need folic acid very early in (at the beginning of) their pregnancy. This means they should start eating healthy **before** they are pregnant.

Women at risk for osteoporosis need to have adequate calcium intakes from their teens through their 40s, a time when their calcium intake is often low.

Because women tend to be smaller than men, they need fewer calories. But they have unique needs related to menstruation, pregnancy, and menopause. Women need to be extra careful to eat nutrient dense foods. That means that they need to get more nutrients per calorie than men.

Five Easy Ideas for Packing Nutrient Dense Foods To Our Diet: Power Packed Eating for Women!
1. Use iron pots to make stews or roasts.
2. Add powdered skim milk to your usual milk or other favorite dishes.
3. Drink calcium fortified juices instead of sodas or other empty calorie beverages.
4. Use evaporated skim milk in enriched and iron fortified hot cereals such as oatmeal.
5. Add soy flakes to dishes such as chili, burgers, or spaghetti sauce.

Seniors

Right now, Latinos are one of the fastest growing segments of the elderly. In this millennium, they will make up a large part of the total U.S. population. Will we be physically, mentally, and financially prepared to retire?

From a nutritional perspective, our energy (calorie) needs decrease about 5 percent per decade of life. So if we needed 2000 calories at age 40, we may only need 1900 calories at age 50, 1805 calories at age 60, and 1715 calories at age 70.

Nutrition related concerns of the older person include dehydration, constipation, lack of appetite, deficiency of Vitamins D, B6, B12, and folate, or the minerals zinc or iron. In our later years, we need to eat more low-calorie, nutrient packed foods. High fiber foods and lots of water intake can help alleviate the common problem of constipation.

We need to avoid a diet of "bread and coffee" or skipping of meals among our elderly. Symptoms of mild malnutrition such as forgetfulness, tiredness, and apathy, may be confused with other diseases. Encourage small, frequent meals that include a variety of foods from all the major food groups.

When should an elderly person be taking supplements? Supplements may be needed if the elderly person is too lonely or sad to eat; taking medications that affect the appetite or the absorption of nutrients; has gastrointestinal illnesses; is losing weight or is immobile. However, you need to discuss this with your doctor and a Registered Dietitian so they can help you determine which supplements are needed and what are the best amounts. Sometimes encouraging the elderly person to go to the local senior citizen's center may provide more benefits than taking dietary supplements.

CONSUMER TIPS

Planning

Identify the health needs of different family members. Start by listing all the things every person can or should be eating. Find the foods you like in common and start your menu plans with that list.

Healthy Snacks for the Entire Family

"All the Time" Snacks
Juices (not ades)
Any fruits
Plain Popcorn
Pretzels
Crackers or bread
Low fat tortilla chips and salsa
Dry unsweetened cereal and low fat milk
Chocolate or strawberry flavored low fat milk
Boiled or baked yams, potatoes, or ripe plantains
Cherry tomatoes
Water packed tuna
"Sometimes" Snacks (Higher Calorie or Fat)
Bread pudding
Rice pudding
Custard or Flan
Peanuts
Sunflower seeds
Pumpkin seeds
Fruit shakes
Cheese—white, cheddar, jack, mozzarella, gouda
A slice of pizza
A hard cooked egg
Sweet breads
A piece of lean cold chicken or turkey

Snacks We Should Eat Infrequently

"Infrequent" Snacks (High Fat, Salt, or Sugar)
Cream cheese
Processed cheese foods or spreads
Meats and fatty cold cuts such as salami, bologna, *chorizo, Vienna sausage*
French fries, fried plantains, or other fried foods
Bread with butter, margarine, or mayonnaise (plain bread is okay)
Doughnuts, cakes
Jelly or honey

ISSUES

Iron-Deficiency Anemia Throughout the Life Cycle

Worldwide iron-deficiency anemia is one of the most common nutrient deficiencies. It occurs mostly in children, teenage girls, women, and less frequently, in teenage males.

In the United States, iron-deficiency anemia sometimes occurs in children because the child drinks too much milk and does not eat enough foods. This is likely to happen if the child is over one year of age and drinking several glasses of milk a day from a baby bottle.

Adolescent girls are going through a growth spurt and, like women, they are losing blood through menstruation. In addition, they may not be getting enough iron-rich foods such as meats or dark, leafy greens. Pregnant women need additional iron for themselves and their baby.

Sometimes adolescent males' rapid growth, high activity levels, increased needs, and erratic eating may cause iron-deficiency anemia.

Eat sources of heme iron (liver, beef, pork, chicken, fish). Drink orange juice or eat high Vitamin C food when you eat the non-heme sources of iron (fortified cereals, beans, dark greens, raisins, peanut butter, etc.). The Vitamin C will help you absorb the iron. Also, cook some of your foods, especially those with tomatoes or tomato sauce, in iron pots.

Anorexia and Bulimia

The eating disorders, anorexia and bulimia, as of yet, are not a very serious health issue for Latinos/Hispanics. However, their consequences can be dangerous and we need to watch for possible symptoms in our loved ones. Females, especially teenage girls, and athletes are most at risk.

A person with anorexia is obsessed with weight loss and refuses to eat. This person may also exercise excessively to promote weight loss. It is important to remember that the weight loss is a *symptom* of other problems—perhaps a desire for perfection, total control, or a distorted perception of self. The person will start to look thin but deny it or try to cover it up by wearing loose clothing.

A person with bulimia eats very large amounts of food then purges—induces vomiting—or abuses laxatives or diuretics. This person will not look thin, as will a person with anorexia, because he or she *is* taking in food. But this distorted eating can cause organ damage, dehydration, and internal bleeding. The teeth may decay from the acids in the vomit. Death may even occur. In both cases, professional intervention is required immediately to prevent serious illness or even death.

CONTEMPORARY LATINO/HISPANIC LIFE

Contemporary Latino life is surrounded with everyday pressures, no matter our age. There are many social changes that make our every day life seem even more hectic, such as the absence of extended families and other support systems. As families try to stay united, it requires extra effort to meet everyone's different nutritional needs.

How can we do this? Here are some easy ideas:

- Occasionally prepare a family member's favorite healthy dish.
- Prepare a basic dish, and at the table, make variations based on family member's special likes or needs.

- Prepare a main dish, and provide side dishes that help meet different family members' special needs.
- Provide different snacks that help meet individual family members' likes and needs.
- Teach family members to make their own special dishes, so the major food preparer can rest once in a while!

Food and Nutrition in This Millennium

As we have additional money to purchase foods and eat out more, obesity, and the related chronic diseases, will become a more serious health issue. There will probably also be an increase in illnesses such as anorexia and bulimia. This increase will be fueled by contemporary pressure for physical beauty. We need to avoid the pressure to measure ourselves against external or material things, and focus on internal beauty and health.

On the positive side, there will be an emphasis on eating foods that promote current and future health. In this millennium, there will be more products designed for special age groups such as infants, children, teens, the elderly, and persons with special health needs. But, do not let advertising have you believe that you **must** buy these special products to eat well. These items may make it easier for you to meet a special need, but you will still be able to eat well by properly selecting non-formulated foods. This millennium will provide an opportunity for all family members to combine traditional and modern foods in ways that are meaningful to each person.

Chapter 10
Managing Your Weight

Introduction

Let's discuss being overweight, its costs and causes. We can go over how to determine if you are overweight. You can then figure out how many calories you need and how many you take in. Then, we can discuss how to set goals and put together a plan for achieving them. Consumer Tips will cover different types of diet plans and provide tips for evaluating them.

General Information

Weight and Body Image. Do you have a friend who thinks that to be beautiful she needs to be tall and thin? Do you have a relative that thinks fat babies are cute? Think about that. These are contradictory values and messages. It seems that advertising glorifies the very tall and thin. But for some cultures, such as Latino/Hispanic culture, being a little heavy has generally been preferred to being thin. So, we are trying to combine these two values. No wonder some of us may feel confused!

What really matters is if we are spiritually, emotionally, and physically fit, and have realistic ideas and goals about our weight. Do you know someone who is thin, but not happy or is unhealthy? How about someone that is always dieting and losing weight only to regain it? Managing our weight is about keeping ourselves physically <u>and</u> emotionally healthy.

Overweight. Many of us are overweight or obese. About one third of the overall US population is overweight. The figures are even higher for Latinos. Among **Latinas,** the highest prevalence of overweight is among women 40-49 years of age. **Latinos'** weights seem to increase as they age. Even if we accept or use more flexible standards, many of us are still overweight.

The Causes of Being Overweight. So why do we gain weight? The more common reason is that we are taking in more calories than we are using up. But there are many "internal" and "external" explanations for why or how this happens. For each of us, the reason for being overweight is probably a combination of these explanations.

Internal explanations include genetics, how many fat cells we produce when we are children, the presence of certain enzymes, our ability to use energy (calories). Also, only about 1% of the obese have a "glandular" problem. While our genes may predispose us to being heavy, it is not the only determinant, and does not doom us to being obese. So, no, don't give up just because your parents were heavy. Doing something will make a difference!

The more common external explanations include overeating and insufficient physical activity. Overeating is often the result of how we react when we see food, and how we act when we are with our family and friends. Do you:

- Prepare or purchase your favorite dish for someone you love (and help the person eat it)?

- Take "eating breaks" or use eating as an excuse for not working or doing something else?

- Find yourself eating more than you want just to please someone else like your Mom, the special date, or your in-laws?

- Look forward to the food at a special party almost as much as, or more than, you look forward to the guests?

- Serve as your family's "garbage disposal" by eating the foods left over on the plates or in the pots and pans?
- Find yourself eating more than you should at a restaurant just to "get your money's worth"?

The Costs of Being Overweight. Obesity costs us time, money, and health. Thinking about how we need to lose weight, how we should do it, and taking steps to lose it, requires a lot of effort. From an economic perspective, in the United States over 5 billion dollars are spent annually on weight reduction products. Over 200 million persons take over-the-counter diet medications. At any point in time, 1/3 to almost 1/2 of persons asked will tell you they are watching their weight. Yet we are getting fatter!

Also, is your weight creating or complicating other health conditions? Excess weight is associated with increased blood pressure, diabetes, high blood cholesterol, hernias, cardiovascular heart disease, and other health conditions. Increased weight aggravates asthma, and may complicate surgery and birthing. Sometimes you can lower your blood pressure by losing a few pounds. If you have type 2 diabetes, you may be able to lower the level of your medications, (maybe not even need them) if you lose weight.

We have about 30-40 billion fat cells that expand to take in extra calories. And, how these fat cells are distributed may put us at higher risk for health problems. Persons that are "apple" shaped are at higher risk than persons that are "pear" shaped. The prevalence of an apple shape is high in Latinos/Hispanics, so we must make extra effort to manage our weight and to care for our health.

If you decide to lose weight, plan to lose it carefully and slowly. The physical instability caused by constantly or quickly gaining and losing weight can be harmful too. If you are going "on and off" diets frequently, this "yo-yo" dieting will be stressful to your body, including your heart.

Determining If You Are Overweight

Three Easy Methods: There are many ways that you can determine if you are overweight. Some ways are easier, and more accurate or appropriate than others. Four easy ones are:

1. Stand in front of the mirror and take a realistic look at yourself. Do you look fat?

2. Stand in front of the mirror and jump up and down. If your body moves more than you want (especially the thighs and stomach), you are flabby and overweight.

3. Determine your waist-to-hip ratio. The easy way to determine your waist-to-hip ratio is to look at your waist (belly) and your hips. If your waist is as big or bigger than your hips (yes…that means your belly is hanging out) you have a high waist-to-hip ratio. The accurate way to determine your waist-to-hip ratio is to measure your waist and measure your hips. Then, divide your "waist" by your "hip." For example, if you are a female and your waist is 30" and your hips are 38": 30/38 = .78 ratio. **A ratio of over .95 for males and .80 for females means that you need to decrease your body fat.**

Compare your weight to a height/weight chart or determine your body mass index. The body mass index is one of the most commonly used methods for determining if a person is overweight or obese. A shortcut way to determine your body mass index is shown in the table below.

Determining Your Body Mass Index		
What to Do	Example	Your Body Mass Index
A. Multiply your weight in pounds by 703	140 X 703 = 98420	
B. Divide the above number by your height (in inches) squared (height x height)	Height = 64 inches height x height = 64 x 64 = 4096	
C. Divide A. by B.	98420/4096 = 24	

Another way to determine your body mass index (BMI) level is to identify your height and weight on a body mass index table, such as the one shown below, which can also be found in http://www.cdc.gov/nccdphp/dnpa/bmi/00binaries/bmi-adults.pdf

Body Mass Index (BMI) Table

BMI	19	20	21	22	23	24	25	26	27	28	29	30	31	32	33	34	35
Height									*Weight (in pounds)*								
4'10" (58")	91	96	100	105	110	115	119	124	129	134	138	143	148	153	158	162	167
4'11" (59")	94	99	104	109	114	119	124	128	133	138	143	148	153	158	163	168	173
5' (60")	97	102	107	112	118	123	128	133	138	143	148	153	158	163	168	174	179
5'1" (61")	100	106	111	116	122	127	132	137	143	148	153	158	164	169	174	180	185
5'2" (62")	104	109	115	120	126	131	136	142	147	153	158	164	169	175	180	186	191
5'3" (63")	107	113	118	124	130	135	141	146	152	158	163	169	175	180	186	191	197
5'4" (64")	110	116	122	128	134	140	145	151	157	163	169	174	180	186	192	197	204
5'5" (65")	114	120	126	132	138	144	150	156	162	168	174	180	186	192	198	204	210
5'6" (66")	118	124	130	136	142	148	155	161	167	173	179	186	192	198	204	210	216
5'7" (67")	121	127	134	140	146	153	159	166	172	178	185	191	198	204	211	217	223
5'8" (68")	125	131	138	144	151	158	164	171	177	184	190	197	203	210	216	223	230
5'9" (69")	128	135	142	149	155	162	169	176	182	189	196	203	209	216	223	230	236
5'10" (70")	132	139	146	153	160	167	174	181	188	195	202	209	216	222	229	236	243
5'11" (71")	136	143	150	157	165	172	179	186	193	200	208	215	222	229	236	243	250
6' (72")	140	147	154	162	169	177	184	191	199	206	213	221	228	235	242	250	258
6'1" (73")	144	151	159	166	174	182	189	197	204	212	219	227	235	242	250	257	265
6'2' (74")	148	155	163	171	179	186	194	202	210	218	225	233	241	249	256	264	272
6'3' (75")	152	160	168	176	184	192	200	208	216	224	232	240	248	256	264	272	279

Source: Evidence Report of Clinical Guidelines on the Identification, Evaluation, and Treatment of Overweight and Obesity in Adults, 1998. NIH/National Heart, Lung, and Blood Institute (NHLBI)

According to the National Center for Health Statistics, a body mass index over 27.3 for women and 27.8 for men is considered overweight. But remember that weight and body mass are not the only indicators of healthy status. There are other factors you want to consider, such as your blood pressure and physical status. It doesn't matter if you are within the designated weight range if you cannot walk just one block without becoming very tired. That means that physically you are probably not very fit.

Identifying Weight Goals

Your Reason(s) for Weight Management. Before you set a numerical weight goal, think about the following: why do you want to lose weight? Have you identified, realistically, whether you are overweight, or would you just like to weigh less? Why? Is it because you feel social pressure to be thin or are unhappy with the way you look? Depending on the reason *why* you want to lose weight, there are factors to consider in order to develop an appropriate plan.

Why Do You Want to Lose Weight?		
Reason You Want to Lose Weight	**Things to Consider**	**Include In Your Weight Management Plan**
To change the way you look.	How you look will largely depend on how you feel about yourself.	Skills on ways to improve appearance, dress.
To have your clothes fit.	Set realistic goals about what fits and your natural body shape.	Some toning exercises.
To be more physically fit.	Merely losing weight will not make you physically fit.	Aerobic and other exercises.
To lower risk for some illnesses (such as diabetes or high blood pressure).	Minimizing risk provides peace of mind, but do not use that as an excuse to ignore regular check-ups.	Learn how to select and prepare foods that help lower the disease risk.

To better manage an illness.	Illness management is important for long term quality of life.	Training in various illness skills such as diet, time, and stress management.
To change your body composition to be leaner, less flabby.	Sometimes you will gain a few pounds because muscle weighs more than fat, but you will look and feel better and be healthier.	Muscle building and toning exercises.
For emotional satisfaction or happiness	Being skinny will not make you happy if you are not happy with yourself. Don't blame emotional unhappiness on excess weight.	Seek professional counseling or care, such as behavior modification to manage foods and emotions.

Weight: Do You Manage It or Does It Manage You? Do you feel hopeless about your weight? Do you know **what, when, where, how, and why** you overeat? You may feel out of control, as though your weight has taken over and you cannot seem to do anything about it.

Remember, it took you a long time to gain the weight. It will take you a while to lose it. To lose it quickly, you have to use dangerous techniques. You will probably regain the weight quickly. Try to lose the weight slowly so you do not feel deprived or either physically or emotionally stressed.

A part of losing weight is to learn new habits you can use once the weight has been lost. That way when you lose the weight, you will have also learned techniques to help you stay that weight.

Some of us think that our weight controls us. We have what is called a fatalistic view about our weight. But, **we have the ability to manage** our weight. If you have identified the causes and reasons for being overweight, you can now work to **figure out ways to successfully** manage your weight.

The Calories In/Out Formula

Estimating Caloric Needs. Do you know why you need the calories? You need calories just for living—that is, for your heart to beat, to think, and for all other body functions (basal metabolism needs). You also need calories for your activities, like walking, cleaning, or cooking (physical activity). To avoid overeating, you need to know the total calories you need for basal metabolism and physical activities.

There are many ways to figure out how many calories you need. If you used each technique, they might give you slightly different ranges, but still a fairly good estimate. One easy way to figure it out is to multiply your weight (in pounds) by 10 if you are a woman, or by 11 if you are a man. Then figure out and add on the activity factor.

Estimating Calorie Needs	
Calculation	Example
Basal needs Multiply your weight by 10 if you are a woman, or by 11 if you are a man.	1. A woman of 130 lbs. 130 X 10 = 1300 basal calorie needs. 2. A man of 160 lbs. 160 X 11 = 1760 basal calorie needs.
Activity factor Multiply your basal calorie needs by one of the following activity factors .20 if you are sedentary. .30 if you have light activity. .40 if you have moderate activity. .50 if you are very active.	1. The woman has light activity—an office job and caring for her 13 year old child: 1300 X .30 = 390 activity calories. 2. The man has a desk job but does exercise about three times a week: 1760 X .40 = 704 activity calories.
Add the basal calorie needs and the activity factor.	1. 1300 + 390 = 1690 her calorie needs. 2. 1760 + 704 = 2464 his calorie needs.

Estimating How Many Calories You Take In. There are four reasons why it is difficult to estimate how many calories you take in. First, because you need to have a general knowledge about the *calorie content of foods.* Second, you need to know *how much you eat.* Third, we tend to *forget* what we eat. And fourth, we tend to *underestimate the amounts* of food we eat.

To estimate how many calories you take in, use the following chart to record what you eat. Do this for at least four days and get an average. Don't change how you eat during those four days, or you will not get accurate data.

Estimate of Food and Calories Eaten

Item (Average calories)	Grain/ Starch (80)	Vegetable (25)	Fruit (60)	Milk/ Dairy (90-150)	Meat/ Substitute (75)	Other* (1 tsp. Oil =50, 1 tbsp. mayo =50, 1 tsp. sugar =25
Example: Tuna sandwich.	2 (160) bread	1/2 cup onions & celery (25)			2 (150)	2 tbsp. mayo (100)
Example: 2/3 ripe plantain, 1 fried egg.	2 (160) plantain				1 (75)	3 tsp. (150) - for frying egg and ripe plantains.
Total Calories	320	25			225	250

Changing the In/Out Balance: No Secret or Magic Formula. There is no secret or magic formula to losing weight. One pound of weight is about 3500 calories. The general formula is that for every 3500 **extra** calories you eat, you will gain about one pound. So, to lose one pound a week you need **to eat 3500 calories less or use up 3500 calories more.** That is about **500 calories per day.**

This may seem like a lot, but it is really not hard to eat 500 calories more than you need per day. A large candy bar or a soda and a small bag of peanuts are almost 500 calories. If you eat one every day, you will have gained one pound in just one week!

Let's think about another example. What if you need 1700 calories a day? You decide to eat about 500 calories at breakfast, lunch, and dinner, and 200 calories for snacks. But you always go to a local restaurant for lunch and have a 2 piece fried chicken combo that is about 900 calories with a soda of 130 calories. If you keep this up, you will be fat within half a year!

How Can You Make These Foods Lower in Fat and Calories?
• Use water packed tuna.
• Use low fat or fat free mayonnaise.
• Use non-stick spray and pan or bake the ripe plantains.
• Use non-stick spray in the pan or poach the egg.

Setting Weight Management Goals

Before you start a weight management plan, be sure to see a physician. Also, ask for a referral to a Registered Dietitian. He or she can help you develop goals and a sound plan.

The safest and more permanent weight loss seems to occur with a weekly loss of about 1-2 lbs. per week. So, if you want to lose 10 lbs., give yourself at least five weeks! If you want to lose 10 pounds for a wedding in June, start a weight management plan around the middle of April.

If you want to lose a large amount of weight, give yourself small goals and continue to add goals. For example, if you need to lose about 50 pounds, first aim for 10 pounds. After you lose them, try for another 10 pounds. This will be achievable and give you small steps to success.

Planning Your Weight Management Program

You can develop a weight management plan. The key is to know how much you need, how much you take in, and how to use the in/out principles.

Three Steps to Planning Your Weight Loss Program
1. Figure out how many calories you need in one day.
2. Adjust in/out formula to meet your goal.
3. Plan menus that will help you follow your in/out plan.

When trying to lose weight, use this formula, but make sure that the total calories taken in are not less than the calories needed for basal needs.

Estimating Calorie Reduction—Sample For A 140 Lb. Woman	
1. Total Calories Needed:	
1400	For basal needs (140 lbs. X 10).
+420	For daily activities (.30 of 1400 for a sedentary life).
=1820	Average total calories needed daily.
2. To Lose About 1 Lb. Per Week:	
1820	Average total calories needed daily.
−500	Calories decreased daily for a weekly 1 lb. weight loss (500 X 7 = 3500).
=1320	Average total calorie diet for weight reduction for a 140 lb. woman.

This person weighs 140 lbs. She should not eat less than 1300 to 1400 calories a day to support basal needs.

Twenty Things You Can Do—Add One of These Each Week!

1. Serve yourself only once.
2. Use a smaller plate.
3. Eat slowly.
4. Only eat—don't do other things while eating.
5. Keep food only in the kitchen.
6. Eat only when hungry, not when bored or tired.
7. Cut away the fat in meat.
8. Use low fat alternatives, like low fat or skim milk.
9. Eat small portions—*meat* no bigger than the palm of your hand or a deck of cards, a piece of *cheese* the size of your thumb, and a serving of rice, pasta, or vegetables the size of a tennis ball.
10. Eat special items you like, but serve yourself one-third to one-half less.
11. Snack on fruits, plain crackers, and calorie free beverages.
12. Eat more fruits and vegetables, less meat, fat, and sugar.
13. Bread and bake foods if you like the "fried" flavor.
14. Balance a high calorie meal with a low calorie meal.
15. Eliminate fat from mixed dishes like in beans, rice, casseroles, soups, and stews.
16. Put more of the low calorie vegetables in soups and stews—less yuca, potato, plantain, sweet potato; more carrots, cabbage, onion, pepper, and tomato.
17. Keep low calorie snacks at home and at work.
18. When you have an appetite, drink water.
19. Identify your "weak moments" and avoid or plan for them.
20. Stop eating before you feel full.

Tips for Managing Your Weight

Certain values and behaviors will help you manage your eating habits. This way of living is beneficial because it is based on preventing becoming overweight. Isn't that **easier** than trying to lose weight?

Easy Ways to Cut Calories. There are many easy ways you can decrease your calories. You don't have to give up good traditional or modern foods, or give up eating out. Ask yourself, how or what would a thin person choose or eat?

Weight Management Tips	
Tip	Example
Focus on fitness and health, not your weight.	• Set a goal to walk 10 blocks instead of a "number on the scale" (No sense in being skinny if you are sickly.)
Intervene early, don't wait until you are very heavy.	• Set yourself an acceptable weight range, like 140 to 145 lbs. • Once you start to weigh 144, go into your weight management action plan.
Incorporate foods you like into your eating plans.	• Plan to eat your favorite guava pastry once a week by including it in your calorie plan. That way you are not taking in **extra** calories when you eat it.
Think about eating healthy for a lifetime, not going on "on and off" diets.	• Eat less for lunch on Friday so you can eat a bit more when you eat out Friday night.
Make activity a regular part of your life.	• Dance *merengue* with the children every day, after dinner, for 1/2 hour.
Have small, manageable goals.	• Replace cola with water as the first weight management goal. • Add another goal to the first goal after one month.
Set a realistic weight goal.	• Lose 1-2 pounds a week, maximum, or start exercising about 20 minutes a day.
Think positive.	• Don't think, "I might as well give up, I can't do it." Think, "How am I going to do this so it can be a part of my life?"

Better yet, observe persons that are thin and healthy, especially among your family and friends. Watch them and see what keeps them thin. What are some of their behaviors? These persons eat only if they are hungry, not just because it is mealtime. They usually serve themselves small amounts of food. Some of them do not like to have a plate that is too full. Some persons are too busy to worry about food because there are other things more important to them than food. For example, they may prefer to go bicycling rather than eating ice cream.

They do not depend on or use food to express love, to share time, to bond, or to reward others. This is hard for us Latinos to do because we love food and it is an important part of our life. We should not use food to "feel better" (as an emotional outlet) or for bonding with others. We can continue to value the importance of food in our life and culture, but we need to remember that it is a vehicle for enjoying relationships, not the center of the relationship.

Exercise. The accepted wisdom about weight management is that a successful plan needs to include some type of activity. This keeps you from needing a very restrictive diet, lets you enjoy more foods, and keeps your body fit.

Ten Exercise Tips

1. Only do a physical activity you like—dancing, walking, bicycling, etc.
2. Exercise at the same time every day.
3. Get an exercise buddy that can help you stay on a routine.
4. Start with a small amount of activity and gradually increase the frequency, time, and intensity.
5. Don't overdo exercise. You'll get too tired or get hurt and quit.
6. Make sure you warm up and cool down.

7. Wear light clothes.

8. Avoid plastic clothes or other gimmicks that make you lose water.

9. Make sure you drink water before, during, and after exercising.

10.Shower after exercising for relaxation and exhilaration.

11.Exercise for at least one half hour while watching television.

CONSUMER TIPS

Evaluating Different Diets and Weight Management Programs

Okay, so how many times have you been on a grapefruit diet? A banana diet? Any other diets? If you have been going on and off diets, chances are that you are now at the weight you wanted to lose when you started going on and off diets. Isn't that depressing? Over the long term, **diets don't work.** And some are worse than others. How can you evaluate an eating plan so that you lose weight, not your money?

First you want to know that there are different types of diets. Within each of these plans there are positive and negative components. What are some types of plans?

Nutrient Focused Plans
Very Low Calorie. Very low calorie diets may be as low as 800 calories. You may see some advertisements for them in magazines, newspapers, or other areas. But these diets can be dangerous because they cause your body muscle to break down, become ketotic, and cause possible damage to your body systems.

You may not feel hungry, but that is not safe. The lack of hunger occurs because the body is (mentally and physically) trying to keep you from *feeling* nutritionally deprived. Because these diets are low in calories, they are also low in the nutrients you need, and deficiencies may result. It is generally not recommended to go on this type of diet. Medically, they are used only in extreme cases and with the close supervision of a doctor, so lab tests can be done and signs of possible harm can be monitored.

Low Carbohydrate, High Protein, or High Fat. You may be told that a low carbohydrate diet is different from a high protein or a low fat diet. Indeed, there are some minor differences. But from a practical perspective, it is hard to have one type of diet without having the other. For example, if you are on a low carbohydrate diet, then the way you will get in food is by either eating high protein, high fat, or high protein and fat. Whenever you decrease one of these calorie-containing nutrients, you are increasing one or both of the other two.

Food Focused Plans

One Food or Limited Foods. How long can you just eat grapefruits? Bananas? Eggs? Cabbage soup? I have seen advertisements for the Lollipop diet, the Wine Lover's diet, and just about every food there is. The reason you generally tend to lose weight on these plans is because you eat less **total** food (**and fewer calories**). Sometimes, as the days go by and you get sick of that food, you eat even less! Of course, you are losing weight because you are probably taking in too few calories and breaking down body tissue. It is not healthy to lose your muscle tissue. And you will gain the weight back once you go off the diet and your body tries to build itself back up.

Some weight loss plans promote the use of a beverage with additional nutrients as a meal replacement. Over short periods of time they are probably not harmful. But, if they are very high in protein, they may be harmful, especially to your kidneys and heart. Generally you will lose a small amount of weight because you have decreased the total calories that you are eating daily. However, these plans generally don't teach you *how to eat the meal you replaced with a beverage.* So, once you have lost the weight, if you go back to eating the same meal, you will probably gain the weight again.

Exchange Plans. In exchange plans, you are given categories of foods and told to select a specific number of servings from the foods in each category. This type of plan was originally designed for persons with diabetes, where the goal was to provide a guideline for regular eating of fixed amounts. When you are given this plan, depending on who wrote it, you may be told that some foods are allowed, not allowed, or free. This is based on the total number of calories that are being planned for you and the calorie ranges of these foods.

The advantage to this plan is that it can help you learn to regulate what you eat and select appropriate serving sizes. If you transfer these behaviors to your everyday life, you will be able to manage weight and food intake. However, you do not have to totally give up foods you like, just include them in the calorie and exchange count. Don't add them on. You won't lose weight if your exchange plan is for 1800 calories and you follow it, but add the ice cream. Make the ice cream (or ice milk) a part of that 1800 calorie limit!

Celebrity or Lifestyle Focused

There can be a wide range of danger or harmfulness to the plan. Do you assume that because your friend is a great computer programmer that he is also an excellent nutritionist? Yet, often we assume that because someone is a famous (maybe not even good person, just famous) that he or she knows about nutrition or exercise.

The celebrity or lifestyle focused plans play on our desire to identify with fame, a characteristic of the person, (usually looks), or the lifestyle. These plans play on our emotions and admiration of others. The next time you see an advertisement for a celebrity diet, or a lifestyle diet (the

Skier's diet, the Swimmer's diet, the Beautiful Model's diet) ask yourself "Is this diet playing on my emotional need or admiration? Is it giving me realistic and sound nutrition advice?"

Behavior Focused Plans

Some of these programs may be called behavior modification, cognitive restructuring, or other terms. Regardless of their name, because their emphasis is on self-awareness and behavior change, they may have good long-term success. However, they generally do not provide "quick fixes" and may be costly.

The DASH (Dietary Approaches to Stop Hypertension) Plan

New research indicates that a diet high in fruits and vegetables (8-10 servings per day) and low fat dairy products (2-3 servings per day) may help with weight loss and management. Although the diet was originally tested to see if it helped decrease high blood pressure (it does), it was also found to help with weight loss and weight management.

Comments

Most weight management programs use a combination of techniques. For example, some may use exchange lists and behavior change. Evaluate their cost, time, likelihood of success (for you), and the professional support that comes with the plan. Check for their nutritional soundness. Does it include *a variety of healthy foods you like to eat, and does not create a dependency on one or a few specific products? Would it be possible for you to eat like this throughout your life?*

ISSUES

Is Dieting Dangerous?

You may have heard some persons say that because dieting is dangerous, it is better to stay fat. The fact is that careful planning and setting realistic goals to change the way you eat will help you lose weight safely. The concern centers on persons that tend to "yo-yo." That is, they gain and lose weight over and over again. This pattern is indeed harmful to the body and not recommended. So don't diet. Develop a sound plan that you can follow for a lifetime.

How About Surgery?

There are various surgical methods available to treat obesity. This includes gastric bypass and gastric stapling for the morbidly obese. Liposuction is also done on the moderately overweight people. However, all these procedures carry different risks. Some procedures may be covered by your medical insurance. Ask your doctor.

CONTEMPORARY LATINO/HISPANIC LIFE

Indeed, in *all* of the Americas, if you want to sell a food, all you have to do is bread it and fry it, and we will eat it! Frying makes food easy to prepare and sell. That is why it is easy to find fried foods anywhere we go.

Eating out is a part of contemporary Latino/Hispanic life. This millennium, it will increasingly become a part of our life. And eating out is no longer limited to "American" fast foods. There are fast food eateries that serve *mofongo, platanos maduros, arroz blanco con frijoles, chifles (mariquitas,* or long, fried, plantain chips) and other traditional Hispanic foods. Like "American" fast foods, the items are often fried, or breaded and fried, or prepared and served with large amounts of fat.

Some Latinos/Hispanics will not go to a fast food restaurant because of the calories in the hamburger and the French fries. Yet, they may go to a restaurant and eat a *biftec empanizado* that is twice the size of their plate (with rice, beans, and tostones, too). Or they will stay home and eat a hamburger that is three times the size of a plain fast food burger. Remember, **it's not where we eat, it's what we eat.**

We can go to a fast food eatery and have a plain burger, salad with fat free dressing, and orange juice. At a fancy restaurant, skip the bread, drink water instead of beer or wine, and take half of that *biftec empanizado, rice, beans, and tostones* home. Eat them as a second meal tomorrow. Moreover, don't feel that you have to eat it all just because you are paying for it.

These eating behaviors will also provide positive examples for your children. They can learn not to eat it all, not to waste food, and ways to save money and be better consumers. Remember, if you feel you have to eat it all just because you paid for it, you are actually paying to **get fat**! Remember, that the *new* diet is the *no* diet…it's **Healthy Lifestyle Choices.**

Food and Nutrition in This Millennium

This millenium there will be greater variety in weight management options. There will be more diet clinics, exercise clubs, weight loss products, pills, and surgical treatments.

The diet of the future will be **no diet**. We have come to realize that diets don't work—for various reasons. First, a diet is something you go "on" and "off." Obviously, going off a diet means that we go back to eating what and how we ate before the diet, which will only get us fat again! Secondly, diets promote a feeling of deprivation, which makes us feel unhappy and desire foods even more. That type of behavior causes overeating.

Weight management programs of the future will try to encourage us to find out why we are overweight and teach us techniques to manage those behaviors. More programs will combine food choices, behavior management, and the other options such as pills or supplements. There will be more programs that combine the "quick" schemes with the more practical and safe approaches. This millennium will belong to the empowered! Managing and caring for your body is your ultimate empowerment!

Chapter 11

Managing Special Diets

General Information

Heart disease. High blood pressure. Diabetes. Cancer. We may have or know someone that has one of these conditions. Do you know what your chances are for getting one of these illnesses? Do you know that how you manage the illness can make a big difference in the quality of your life? Would you be ready, willing, and able to do some of the things that will help minimize a disease's progress and complications? Can you go to a food store or restaurant and select foods that you enjoy that also help you manage your condition?

This chapter will cover some basic information about heart disease, high blood pressure, diabetes, and cancer. The section on Consumer Tips will provide information about shopping and eating out that may help you prevent or manage your condition.

Heart Disease

Most of us know that heart disease is the major cause of death for men. But did you know that heart disease is also the major cause of death for women? Heart disease is a major killer of most Latinos. But there is much we can do to prevent heart disease. With just a few lifestyle changes, we can increase our chances of having a healthy heart.

Heart disease is a general term that covers many different types of heart related diseases. Heart disease can also be caused by irregular heartbeats or valve related problems. Arteriosclerosis is hardening of the arteries and atherosclerosis is clogging of the arteries.

Arteriosclerosis and atherosclerosis occur over time. Although we do not know exactly how or why, smoking, high blood pressure, and high blood cholesterol are risk factors. Tobacco products seem to injure the linings and the smoke seems to increase plaque buildup in the arteries. High blood pressure puts an additional strain on the heart.

Heart disease is a life altering condition. Prevention and treatments of choice involve lifestyle changes such as diet, exercise, and stress management. The most common and easily applied recommendations are to eat less fat and salt, to avoid smoking, to increase physical activity, to develop positive approaches to managing life's stresses, and to include relaxation and spiritual wellness activities.

What Do HDL, LDL and High Blood Cholesterol Mean?

You may have heard of high blood cholesterol. The level of 200mg/dl is the commonly used "alarm" level. Or, you may have been tested for your HDL or LDL levels. HDL, or high-density lipoproteins, are believed to help carry cholesterol away from the cells and help keep the arteries clear. So, it is desirable to have a high HDL level (greater than 40mg/dl; even higher is better for women). Low-density lipoproteins, or LDLs, are believed to carry cholesterol, and promote their settling into the arteries. So, it is desirable to have a low LDL level (less than 100mg/dl).

> • Do you exercise? Did you know that it helps raise your HDL levels?
> • Do you eat beans, oatmeal, and soups or dishes made with high fiber vegetables?
> **If you do, you are on your way to a healthy heart!**

Many persons believe that the way to have a healthy heart is to eat fewer foods with cholesterol (like lard, bacon, fatty beef or pork, fried skins, cheese, whole milk, butter, cream cheese, red or fatty meats, and eggs). While it is important to cut down on these cholesterol-containing foods, it is **more important** to cut down on the **total** amount of fats (and especially the saturated fats) in the diet. So, it is also important to eat less coconut, margarine, and other hydrogenated fats. Although the polyunsaturated (like corn oil) and the monounsaturated fats (like olive oil, or the fat in avocado and peanuts) are beneficial, it is still important to only eat them in small amounts.

If you have heart disease, your treatment will depend on the type of heart disease you have, and other factors and conditions. In general, treatment may consist of a special diet, exercise, medications, and in more advanced or serious situations, some type of surgery.

Healthy Heart Choices	
Recommendations	Examples
Eat more fruits, vegetables, whole grains, legumes, low fat dairy products.	Orange, pineapple, mango, sweet potatoes, *yautia, mamey, watercress,* whole wheat tortillas, oatmeal, *atole* beverage*(of oatmeal), mango shake,* beans, and low fat milk.
Use monounsaturated or polyunsaturated fats.	Olive oil, avocado, nuts, safflower oil, canola oil, sunflower oil, corn oil, **in small amounts.**
Avoid foods high in saturated fats.	Coconut, coconut oil, lard, bacon, fatty beef or pork, fried "skins," cheese, whole milk, butter, margarine, hydrogenated fat (frying fats), cream cheese, canned meats, red or fatty meats.
Eat less sodium and salt.	Use fresh fruits, vegetables, and meats. Avoid canned foods, quick or instant foods, cured meats or cold cuts, salted and dried fish, salty snacks, ketchup.

High Blood Pressure

High blood pressure is another common illness among Latinos. Many of us think that our blood pressure only gets "high" when we are upset or annoyed. But high blood pressure happens when our vessels

have become stiff and/or narrow, and not from social tension that we
feel when we are angry or upset. When our vessels have become stiff
and/or narrow, the blood must work harder than usual to pass through
our vessels. This extra "pushing" damages the heart walls and may be
occurring even though we may not be feeling it. Yes, some social situations can cause our blood pressure to rise. But, in general, high blood
pressure is not something we feel as we go about our daily life.

We may have high blood pressure and not know it. It is important to
get blood pressure checks regularly, especially if we have relatives with
that condition. A United States study found that about 25% of Mexican
American men, 22% of Cuban men, and over 15% of Puerto Rican men
have high blood pressure. Over 20% Mexican American, 15% of Cuban,
and 11% of Puerto Rican women have high blood pressure.

Are you in the *undiagnosed* group? Untreated high blood pressure can
damage our heart, kidneys, and other organs, even though we are not
"feeling it." If we are "feeling it," then it has become *very* serious and we
are having complications. Don't let it get this far before you take action!

How is blood pressure measured?

There are two numbers used to measure your blood pressure. The
desirable reading is 120/80. The "120," or the top number, is the systolic
number. This is your pressure when the heart contracts to pump out
blood. The "80" or the bottom number, is the diastolic pressure. This is
your pressure when the heart is at rest. If you are in the 130-139/85-89
range, your pressure is "high normal" and you need to get it checked
regularly. A blood pressure reading at or above 140/90 is high and we
need to work with the doctor to control this high level.

The good news is that there are many things we can do to manage
our high blood pressure. Among them:

• If we are overweight, we can lose weight.

• If we smoke, we can stop smoking.

- We can eat less salt or sodium and more high calcium, low fat foods.
- If we drink, we must avoid excessive drinking (not more than one drink a day or less).
- We can eat a diet high in fruits and vegetables (8-10 servings per day) and low fat dairy products (2-3 servings per day), which seem to help not only with decreasing high blood pressure, but also with weight loss and management.
- We can do some, or more, exercise.

Diabetes

In this book we have talked about blood sugar (glucose), and how it is the fuel that gives us energy. Let's look at how that is related to diabetes. Insulin, which is made in our pancreas, helps us regulate and use our blood sugar (glucose). If we do not make any or enough insulin, we cannot use this energy. As a result, the glucose builds up in our blood, and we have trouble controlling blood sugar levels, and have "high blood sugar."

There are three types of diabetes. Type 1 usually starts when the person is a child and cannot make any, or enough, insulin. Type 2 diabetes often runs in families and generally begins in mid-adult life. Gestational diabetes occurs in some women when they are pregnant. It disappears after the baby is born, but may reappear later in life.

Did you know that more than 1 in 10 (1.8 million) Hispanic adults have type 2 diabetes? And it is estimated that another half don't know they have diabetes and are undiagnosed! Because the prevalence of type 2 diabetes is high in Hispanics, **we must take special care** to prevent and treat it.

Latinos, especially Mexican-Americans and Puerto Ricans, are at high risk for type 2 diabetes. Although diabetes is lower in Cuban Americans, it is still considered high. For Latinos 45 to 74 years old, about 26 percent of Puerto Ricans, 24 percent of Mexican-Americans, and 16 percent of Cuban Americans have diagnosed diabetes.

We are especially at risk if we have relatives with diabetes, if we are over 40 years old, or are obese (particularly around our central upper body, the belly). Although the rate of diabetes is lower in Latinos ages 20 to 44, this is an important age in which to avoid getting too fat. Controlling your weight during this period may help to avoid diabetes, delay its onset, or help with its management.

We are also at risk if we have high blood pressure or high blood cholesterol levels, if we have had high blood sugar levels, or had gestational diabetes. Urine tests should be done as part of your regular physical exam. An impaired glucose tolerance test (IGT) can help determine if we are in an early stage of diabetes.

Possible signs or symptoms of diabetes include blurred vision, fatigue, infections or cuts that do not heal, hunger, frequent urination, and thirst. The excess sugar in the blood affects vision. We feel tired because we are not using sugar effectively for energy. The high blood sugar does not let the body use the nutrients needed for healing. The body has to get rid of the extra sugar, so we urinate a lot. That makes us thirsty. However, sometimes a person with diabetes may *feel no symptoms*, so it is important to get checked regularly.

Managing diabetes is very important because of the seriousness of its complications. These can include damage to the kidneys, eyes, and blood vessels. Poor circulation can lead to amputations. To manage diabetes, take the pills or insulin injections regularly, if they have been prescribed. You need to regulate the amount of carbohydrates you eat by using exchange diets or counting carbohydrates. This will help you eat the right amounts of foods regularly, which in turn will help the body have a constant and correct amount of energy, and a stable amount of blood sugar. This will serve to prevent some of the complications that occur from the blood sugar levels going too high or too low. A Registered Dietitian (RD) can help you develop an eating plan.

Cancer

There are many types of cancers. Cancer of the lung is the leading cause of cancer death in both sexes. Although it is lower in Latinos than in some other groups, it is still high. Lung cancer is higher in males than females, especially those 30-54 years old.

Cancer of the cervix is one of the common types of cancer among women. It is especially important that women get regular check-ups if they are between 30-69 years old. Early diagnosis and treatment increases the chances of a good outcome. Breast cancer is higher in women that are obese, never had children, or live in urban areas.

Dietary factors and exercise appear to be very important in the prevention of colorectal cancer. The rates of colorectal cancer decrease as we become more physically active and eat less fats, fatty meats, and fried foods.

CONSUMER TIPS

Heart Disease

If you are at risk for, or have heart disease, remember the following when eating out or shopping:

- Vegetable, thin crust, and whole wheat pizzas are generally healthier and **lower in sodium** than three cheese, pepperoni, sausage, anchovy, or olive topped pizzas.

- Fried foods are high fat.

- White sauces (like Alfredo sauce, coleslaw) are high in fat.

- Dressings, especially "creamy dressings" (like creamy Italian, Blue Cheese or Ranch) are high in saturated fat.

- A salad with a large packet of regular dressing may have as much or more fat than a lean plain burger or a plain grilled chicken sandwich.
- Pick low fat or low calorie dressings.

High Blood Pressure

If you have high blood pressure, remember the following when eating out or shopping:

- Fresh fruits, vegetables, and meats tend to be lower in salt or sodium than instant or pre-prepared foods.
- Ask that your foods be prepared without salt, and do not add any at the table.
- Large amounts of sodium or salt are found in processed foods, such as canned, instant, dried, and cured foods.
- Some sweet foods, like ketchup, are high in sodium.
- Most commercial seasonings are high in salt.

Take your blood pressure medication, even if you do not feel that your blood pressure is high.

There Is A Big Difference In Sodium Levels!			
Sodium In Fresh Product		Sodium In Processed Product	
Fresh Product	Sodium in Milligrams	Processed Product	Sodium in Milligrams
1 cup regular oatmeal.	2	3/4 cup instant oatmeal.	286
1 fresh baked potato.	16	1/2 cup mashed potato, made from flakes.	349
3–1/2 oz. lean ground beef.	56	3 1/2 oz. canned corned beef.	1006
1 cup boiled pinto beans.	3	1 cup canned pinto beans.	998
1/2 cup boiled yellow corn.	14	1/2 cup canned yellow corn.	286
1 fresh apple with skin.	1	1/6 apple pie.	195

Diabetes

If you have diabetes, remember the following when eating out or shopping:

- Portion size is important. Try to get foods that are close to your recommended serving sizes. The "super size" may be a better price but **not** be a better choice for you.
- Sugar-free does not mean calorie-free or healthy for you. Sugar-free foods may still have honey, fructose, sorbitol, or other sugars, sugar substitutes, or fat. Include these calories in your eating plan.
- Eating regularly is important for you. Buy high fiber and whole wheat snacks you can carry if you will not be near an eatery at meal or snack times.

Cancer

To prevent some cancers it is recommended that we eat more of the following:

- Cruciferous vegetables like cabbage and brussel sprouts.
- Fruits and vegetables with dark orange or red colors, like mangoes, papaya, and tomatoes.
- Soy based products like soymilk or tofu.

ISSUES

There are three important issues related to these conditions that we need to be aware about:

- Prevention behaviors.
- Early diagnosis and treatment.
- Management and control of disease progress.

We can take charge of our lives and do things that help prevent or delay getting heart disease, diabetes, hypertension, or cancer. In addition, for some Latinos, the condition is made worse if we do not find out about the illness early. As a result, we miss the opportunity and steps that can be taken to manage the illness and prevent complications.

CONTEMPORARY LATINO/HISPANIC LIFE

As you can see, there are some similar or common recommendations for these illnesses. For example: losing weight, exercising, cutting fats or extra calories, and avoiding excessive amounts of sugar or salt. Making a few changes can help you decrease the risk for, or better manage, one or several conditions.

Add More Flavor—Not More Fat or Salt!

- Sauté your onions in chicken broth instead of oil, and put them over boiled *yuca* or green bananas.
- Make your own *adobo* or seasoning mixes. Mix black and white pepper, dried coriander (*cilantro*), cumin, garlic powder, and other favorite seasonings.
- Use yellow food coloring instead of annato (*achiote*) oil.
- Add more *cilantro* or Italian seasoning mix (oregano, parsley, and basil) and less salt to tomato based dishes and your favorite stews.
- Marinate meats in homemade low salt *adobo* and a fancy vinegar or lemon juice, and skip the oil. Traditional beans, fruits, vegetables, and small amounts of olive oil are healthy for us.
- Use undiluted evaporated milk, cinnamon, and/or vanilla instead of butter to flavor your hot cornmeal, oatmeal, mashed ripe plantains and pumpkin.
- Use garlic, pepper, and undiluted evaporated milk instead of butter and salt in your mashed potatoes.
- Slice potatoes and sprinkle them with homemade low salt *adobo* and bake!

Food and Nutrition in This Millennium

Developments in human genetics and the impact of lifestyle on health will help us identify our potential risk for various diseases. This millennium we will be able eat to "eat for our genes" and use information about our genetics to decrease our risk for disease. There will be more information on ways to combine healthy eating, exercise, new medications, and "alternative" treatments. There will also be an emphasis on learning relaxation and other stress management techniques.

Chapter 12
Eating Out, Snacking, and Holiday Eating

General Information

If you worry about managing your weight or about the eating habits of your loved ones, then it is important to know the following:

- Hispanics in the United States eat more fast food and drink more colas than other groups.

- An important component to managing weight is selecting low calorie foods when eating out, snacking, and eating holiday foods.

- More people are snacking throughout the day instead of eating three full meals.

- It is estimated that people gain an average of two to five pounds during the fall holiday season.

Foods that we eat out and many of our snacks and holiday foods are high in fat, salt, and sugar. For example, sometimes eating a popular presweetened cereal is almost like eating a candy bar. If you combine this with drinking one or two sodas throughout the day, it is easy to see how we are consuming too much sugar! The popular potato chip and soda snack is almost like having a snack of **salt and sugar!**

Eating Out

In general, people are eating out more. The biggest increase in eating out has occurred among women and children. This is probably related to women entering the workforce and the increased number of children in childcare.

More than half of Americans eat outside the home at least once a day. But some persons may be eating out two or more times a day. For example, some persons have breakfast in the car and lunch at work, or, eat lunch out and eat out again on the way home. If the person buys a mid-afternoon snack, that would add up to eating out three times in one day.

Latinos are more likely than other Americans to buy food out and bring it home. But whether we eat it out or bring it home, it is important to remember that unless we select carefully, we will likely be bringing home foods high in fat, calories, and salt. The key to bringing foods home is to balance what is brought home with nutritious side dishes added from home.

Snacking

Snacking is now a way of life for many persons. It can be a very effective way to manage your weight, provide quick energy, or fill up on missing nutrients. Snacking puts less stress or load on the heart, and is less likely to cause heartburn than a big meal.

Snacks can make up 1/5 or more of our total calories, especially for pre-school children and teenagers. Snacks can be very costly. Purchase or prepare snacks that will provide lots of nutrients for the money, and try to have them easily and quickly available.

Holiday Eating

Holiday time is a fun time. So, in general, this is not the time to deprive yourself of your favorite foods. It's hard to have fun if you are feeling deprived. Focus instead on making the recipes healthier by adding more vegetables and using less sugar or fat. Eat smaller amounts of food and try to move around more.

What are your favorite holiday foods? For most Latinos roast pork is a popular holiday food. Various versions of tamales or the Puerto Rican *pastel* (green plantain and pork dish) may be prepared as part of a family tradition. For dessert, the family favorites may include rice or bread puddings, *Flan*, *habichuelas con dulce* (sweet beans), *churros* (crullers) or *buñuelos* (beignets), or various types of cakes. Many of these dishes can be made with 1/3 – ½ less fat or sugar, or they can be baked instead of fried.

CONSUMER TIPS

Snacking

When trying to select a snack, try to have one or two items from the basic groups of the Food Guide Pyramid. Because taste is the primary reason why people choose a snack, make sure it is something healthy that you enjoy eating!

What Can You Do to Eat Well While at Work?

- Anticipate. Buy low calorie snacks such as baked potato chips or plain popcorn and keep them by the door at home. Grab one on the way to work.

- Keep small cans of juices and bottles of water at work. This helps you drink the water you need, increase the intake of fruits, and decrease intake of less nutritious items such as soda and coffee throughout the day.

- Keep crackers, pretzels, popcorn, bananas, apples, or low calorie snack items at work. This will help avoid the temptation of buying high fat and high calorie snacks such as doughnuts or chips when you want a snack that you can chew.

- Keep small cans of milk or powdered milk at work for coffee or hot chocolate. Half and half and other creamers are high in fat and contain little or no calcium.

- Eat a healthy snack before you leave work so that you are not tempted to eat high fat or high calorie snacks on the way, or once you get home.

Suggested Beverages	Suggested Snacks
Water (plain or flavored, without sugar)	Unsalted soda or whole wheat crackers
Orange juice	Low fat or baked tortilla chips
Grapefruit juice	Vanilla wafers
Pineapple juice	Peanuts
Apricot nectar	Pretzels (unsalted are best)
Tomato juice	Popcorn (low fat or fat free)
Vegetable juice	Small cans of tuna or salmon without added fat
Mixed fruit juices (100% juice)	Small cans of vegetables

How Can I Make Dry Cereals A Healthy Snack Food?

- Purchase dry cereal that has some fiber, about three grams or more per serving.

- Select a dry cereal with a moderate amount of sugar, about four to six (1-1/2 teaspoons) per serving.

- Make a cereal mix with different dry cereals, nuts, and dried fruit. Put the mix in small plastic bags for easy grabbing.

- Serve the small bag of dry cereal with a glass of milk, juice, or water.

Did You Know that About 4 Grams Equals One Teaspoon?
If your cereal says 16 grams of sugar for a one-cup serving, it's as if you had put four teaspoons of sugar in your cup of cereal!

Eating Out

There are several points to consider when eating out:

- Does the eatery offer both low and higher calorie choices?
- Is there a range of portion sizes?
- Are you likely to overeat in that food setting?
- Can you easily share a meal? (Share a meal and eat fewer calories!)
- You have a right to ask for a modification, for example, broiled instead of fried, dressing or sauce on the side, to share a dish, or a bag to take food home.

Holiday Eating

Preplanning

At least one month before the holiday season, start practicing some control behaviors and preparing yourself for the holidays. For example:

- Start doing a small amount of extra exercise.
- Practice modifying some of the holiday recipes to make them lower in fat and calories.
- Start serving yourself smaller portions of food so you get used to eating smaller meals.
- Start drinking water and drinking other calorie-free or low-calorie drinks that you can request at parties so you can get used to their flavor (like water with a lime, a diet ginger ale with a lemon wedge, etc.).
- Imagine scenarios where food is in abundance and practice ways to avoid overeating (for example, how you might select certain foods, how you will carry around the diet cola to keep your hands too busy to grab other snacks, or where you will stand so you are not near the food table, etc.)

Going to the Celebration

The key to avoiding gaining weight is to focus on the company and the non-eating activities, and to plan ways to use up the extra calories.

• Try to do at least ten minutes of exercise before you get dressed and ready to leave. Or do some extra housework (do the wash, sweep the floors, etc.) that uses lots of calories.

• Drink something that will fill you up just before you leave the house, such as a glass of low fat milk. Make sure you do not leave the house hungry.

• As you walk into the party remind yourself that the fun is in the talking, dancing, socializing, not the eating or the drinking.

• Make the first thing you have at the party at least two glasses of a calorie-free beverage.

• Give yourself a limit of one. For example, one glass of wine mixed with ginger ale, one of the best appetizers. Focus on quality, not quantity.

• Always keep your hands busy holding a calorie-free beverage on one hand and a low-calorie food on the other (like a carrot stick).

• Have the plain raw vegetables instead of the chips.

• Have the salsa instead of the cream based dips.

• Scrape the frosting away from the desserts.

• Once you feel slightly full, put a dirty napkin on your plate to prevent yourself from picking on more food.

• Don't bring any food home, unless it's the low calorie vegetables.

Three Ways to Say "no" Nicely
1. Tell them it tastes delicious, but you are already very full.
2. Tell them it was so good that you want to take the rest home.
3. Tell them you want to taste other foods and are saving some "space."

After the Party

• Go home and drink water before going to bed. Do not eat food again.

• Do some extra exercise the next day. Park farther away from work; use the stairs instead of the elevator, etc.

• Eat small meals. Have a small breakfast and dinner, or have no meats or fats. Avoid any fried or high calorie foods.

• Have water, fruit, or skim milk as a snack.

ISSUES

Feed the Physical Not the Social or Emotional Needs

For some of us, eating is more of a social or emotional act than a physiological act. As a result, we eat not because we are hungry, but because:

• We enjoy both being with and sharing food with other people.

• We want to impress someone (like taking someone to an expensive restaurant).

• We are using food to demonstrate a "status" (like bringing in an expensive or new beverage to work).

• We are trying to compensate for other needs (like eating because we are lonely, angry, or sad).

• We are trying to substitute a negative or boring routine with a more pleasant activity (like snacking to relieve stress or get a break from answering the phones at work).

• We feel social pressure to eat (like during the holidays, when your mother spent hours making that high calorie cake).

CONTEMPORARY LATINO/HISPANIC LIFE

Imagine the following scenarios. They are fairly common, and we need to be careful not to fall into these "eating traps":

Scene 1
You do not want to go to a fast food restaurant because you feel it has many high calorie foods. Instead you go to a restaurant. But while you are waiting for the meal, you have bread and/or a salad with lots of dressing. You order a steak that is much bigger than a three or four-ounce burger, and you have one of the fancy desserts!

Scene 2
You do not want to go to a fast food restaurant, because you feel it has many high calorie foods, or because you feel it is a costly activity. Instead, you purchase some ground beef at the supermarket. You go home and make everyone homemade burgers and fries. But, because you do not like those "small burgers," the ones you make at home are actually about 6 or more ounces, much bigger and fatter than the ones you would have eaten out!

Scene 3
You go to an all-you-can-eat restaurant because you feel it has more variety than other eateries. But in addition to the salad, you eat many of the items, so you can feel like you are getting your money's worth!

How might you handle these situations?

Scene 1
Go to fast food places, instead of restaurants, if you eat out often. They tend to be less expensive. Select the low fat and low calorie options. For example:

- Have a plain regular burger or plain grilled chicken, a small side salad, and a glass of juice.
- Order one or two soft tacos, and a glass of low fat milk or juice.
- Have the ham and cheese, or plain turkey sandwich, with a glass of milk or juice.
- Have the chicken or chef's salad with low calorie or fat free dressing, a glass of low fat milk or juice, and the crackers. Skip the croutons!
- Have the children's meal, if allowed.

But, if you choose to go to a restaurant:

- Tell them not to bring you bread (or the butter) before the meal.
- Drink water to fill yourself up.
- Have a small side salad with low calorie dressing on the side.
- Order the smallest piece of meat available.
- Eat only half the meal and share the other half or take it home with you.
- Eat the rest as a second meal.
- Skip dessert or have plain coffee with low fat milk.

Scene 2

- Purchase lean turkey and beef (or soybean flakes) at the supermarket.
- Make a burger mix and measure your burgers so they are no more than 3-4 ounces (like the size of a deck of cards).
- Serve with sliced, herb seasoned, baked potatoes.
- Make a homemade orange drink using fresh juice, water, and sugar substitute.
- Serve with a nice fresh fruit salad.

Scene 3

Go to the all-you-can-eat restaurant and:

- First serve yourself a big salad with lots of greens, tomatoes, mushrooms, carrots, and peppers and low calorie dressing.
- Then, fill the plate with vegetables (like broccoli, green beans, boiled cabbage or leafy greens and vegetable medley) and just one very small piece of a meat, poultry, or fish.
- Then, serve yourself fruit salad.
- If you want something special, put a small amount of the ice cream on top of the fruit salad.
- Stop eating before you feel full!

Food and Nutrition in This Millennium

Eating out is one thing that we will all continue to do more, so it is important to become wise consumers and learn to select healthy, low calorie foods away from home. Develop some eating out strategies. These should include:

- A technique for quickly comparing "price for value" at different eateries.

- A family plan and schedule for eating at the more expensive restaurants, such as combining two family members' birthdays or providing a choice between eating out or a gift.

It is important to develop and teach these strategies to your children. After all, as they continue to prosper in this millennium, these consumer skills will be used and carried on to other activities.

Chapter 13
Putting It All In Perspective

Introduction

Many years ago someone asked me what my favorite foods were. I responded rice, beans, Chinese egg rolls, knishes, pizza, and many other foods. I still remember the confused look on her face when I named foods that are not part of my traditional culture. But all the foods mentioned are a part of me! Liking and eating non-traditional as well as traditional foods does not minimize, and is not a negation of, a person's cultural identity.

This millennium will provide all of us with even more opportunities to eat traditional and modern foods, and every combination in between. This chapter will provide some menus that are based on the information in this book. The menus include typical foods, new foods, foods of other cultures, and ideas for fast foods you can make or buy.

The menus are just guides for how to select and/or prepare healthy foods, no matter your goals or where you are. My hope for you is your knowledge that all foods, and the right choices that you make, can enable you to live a healthy life.

SAMPLE MENUS

Breakfast—at Home or on the Road

Breakfast is, and will continue to be, one of the most important meals of the day. The menus included here are designed to give you ideas for eating at home or eating on the run. Many of these items can be made quickly in advance, or purchased already prepared. Some of these foods can be taken along or carried in one hand, if necessary, or eaten leisurely while enjoying the company of your loved ones.

Choice 1	Choice 2	Choice 3	Choice 4	Choice 5
Grilled cheese sandwich (with whole wheat bread and two tomato slices) Coffee with low fat milk	One scrambled egg (with chopped peppers and onions) in two corn tortillas Coffee with low fat milk	Bran flakes or oat cereal with low fat milk Banana Coffee with low fat milk	One cup oatmeal (made with low fat milk) Mixed berry juice (100% fruit juice) Coffee with low fat milk	Sesame seed bagel Two tablespoons of peanut butter Orange juice Coffee with low fat milk
Choice 6	Choice 7	Choice 8	Choice 9	Choice 10
French Toast or pancake topped with canned peaches Coffee with low fat milk	*Atole* (made with *masa harina*, sugar, cinnamon and low fat milk) or instant breakfast drink Apple	One cold broiled chicken leg One slice Italian bread 10 grapes Coffee with low fat milk	Ham sandwich (on English Muffin) Dried papaya Coffee with low fat milk	¼ cup egg substitute, scrambled ¼ cup white rice ¼ cup black beans Coffee with low fat milk

Lunch Away From Home

Choice 1	Choice 2	Choice 3	Choice 4	Choice 5
Plain cheeseburger and side salad or a grilled chicken salad. Low calorie dressing Small orange juice	1 ½ cups canned hearty vegetarian soup One slice Italian bread One small piece of cheese 1 glass vanilla flavored soymilk	Sliced turkey, cheese, lettuce, and tomato sandwich (on whole wheat bread) Apple juice	1 ½ cups homemade chicken soup with potato, carrots, green peppers, onions, cilantro One slice French bread Spanish decaffeinated coffee with low fat milk	One slice pizza with peppers and onions and a side salad with low calorie dressing Mixed juice (100% fruit juice)
Choice 6	**Choice 7**	**Choice 8**	**Choice 9**	**Choice 10**
Arepa (with a small amount of cheese) Fruit Smoothie	Chinese stir fry vegetables with white rice Iced Tea	Two ounces of tuna Roll Mixed fruit salad Pineapple juice	6" Vegetarian sandwich Strawberry or other flavor low fat milk	Boiled *yuca* Three to four lean roast pork cubes (*masitas*) *Mamey* fruit shake (*batido*)

Dinners as Diverse as Our Preferences

Choice 1	Choice 2	Choice 3	Choice 4	Choice 5
Chicken and rice (1 cup rice, 3 oz. chicken) ½ cup peas Sliced tomatoes with vinegar and basil Apple juice spritzer*	Vegetarian spaghetti (1 cup spaghetti sauce made with textured soy vegetable protein 1 ½ cups pasta, ¼ cup shredded fat-free cheese) One slice Italian bread Tossed salad with low calorie dressing Water	Gazpacho Three ounces breaded, oven baked fish Three *tostones* Caesar salad Diet lemonade	Two-three soft corn tacos with Ground beef and textured soy vegetable protein mix, lettuce, tomato, onion, shredded cheese Pineapple juice	One baked lean pork chop Tossed salad with lettuce, cabbage, tomatoes, carrots, and avocado with vinegar ½ cup white rice Fruit juice spritzer*
Choice 6	Choice 7	Choice 8	Choice 9	Choice 10
One cup Chinese Fried rice Steamed chicken or tofu and vegetables Hot tea	Two bean and cheese burritos Tomato slices with vinegar One glass orange juice	One cup yellow rice ½ cup Spanish style stewed ground beef (*picadillo*) Tossed green salad with low fat dressing Decaffeinated coffee with low fat milk	Spanish Omelet (egg substitute, potato, onion, tomato, shredded fat free cheese) One cup green beans Two slices French bread Diet soda or water	One cup white rice One cup *Feijoada* (Brazilian black beans made with turkey sausage) Cucumber, tomato, and onion salad Fresh fruit drink

• Mix equal parts juice and diet ginger ale or seltzer water

CONSUMER TIPS

There are many places that you can go for information. Some of these are in your own community, others you can access without ever leaving your home.

Local

If you have nutrition related questions call the local:

- hospital or public health department and ask to speak to a licensed nutritionist or Registered Dietitian;
- universities and ask if they have nutrition professors that you can speak with;
- state university to see if they have a "Cooperative Extension" office. Ask for the home economics, nutrition, or family and consumer sciences specialist;
- City Hall and ask for the Department of Consumer Affairs.

On-line

You may also get some useful nutrition information on the Internet from various non-profit organizations or food companies. But be careful. Remember, many sites have inaccurate or misleading information, and some organizations or companies are trying to sell you their products or have an agenda that may not be in your best interest or health! Here are some sources that provide reliable nutrition information:

American Cancer Society http://www.cancer.org/
American Diabetes Association http://www.diabetes.org/main/community/outreach/latinos/default2.jsp
American Dietetic Association http://www.eatright.org/
American Heart Association http://www.americanheart.org/

CDC en Español (Centers for Disease Control) http://www.cdc.gov/spanish/default.htm
La Leche League International http://www.lalecheleague.org/
American Institute for Cancer Research http://www.aicr.org/
National Heart, Lung and Blood Institute http://www.nhlbi.nih.gov/health/prof/heart/latino/latin_pg.htm
Office of Dietary Supplements http://ods.od.nih.gov/index.aspx
Office of Minority Health http://www.omhrc.gov/omhrc/
The Vegetarian Resource Group http://www.vrg.org/
United States Department of Agriculture http://www.nal.usda.gov:8001/py/pmap.htm http://www.nal.usda.gov/fnic/etext/000023.html#xtocid2381818 (link to Puerto Rican, Latin American, Mediterranean, Spanish, and other Food Guide Pyramids and the Dietary Guidelines)
National Council of La Raza http://www.nclr.org/policy/health.html

Food and Nutrition in This Millennium

This millennium will bring us more choices, places, and new foods to eat than have ever been available. New developments in the health sciences, nutrition, and genetics will help us identify early diet related diseases for which we may be at high risk. This means that we will have more choices and also more control over our health. That is a great opportunity for a healthy life. Here's wishing you a healthy appetite, wise food choices, and great health!

Reader Survey

Please provide us with your ideas for future books by responding to the following questions:

What did you like most about *Contemporary Nutrition for Latinos?*

1. _____
2. _____

What did you like least about *Contemporary Nutrition for Latinos?*

1. _____
2. _____

What would you like in future publications about foods, nutrition and Latinos?

1. _____
2. _____
3. _____
4. _____

Please mail to:
Dr. Judith C. Rodriguez
UNF/COH/DPH
4567 St. Johns Bluff Rd. So.
Jacksonville, FL 32224

Additional copies of this book can be
obtained at www.iuniverse.com.

0-595-29730-7

Printed in the United States
20210LVS00007B/1-78